JOHANNA BURANI, M.S., R.D., C.D.E.
LINDA RAO, M.ED.

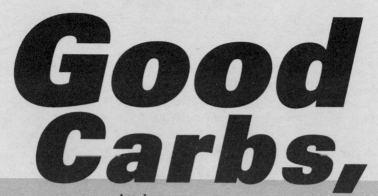

Good Carbs,

AN INDISPENSABLE
GUIDE TO EATING THE RIGHT CARBS
FOR LOSING WEIGHT AND OPTIMUM HEALTH

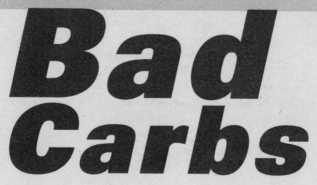

Bad Carbs

MARLOWE & COMPANY
NEW YORK

GOOD CARBS, BAD CARBS:
*An Indispensable Guide to Eating the Right Carbs
for Losing Weight and Optimum Health*
Copyright © 2002 by Johanna Burani and Linda Rao

Published by
Marlowe & Company
An Imprint of Avalon Publishing Group Incorporated
161 William Street, 16th Floor
New York, NY 10038

Library of Congress Cataloging-in-Publication Data
Burani, Johanna C.
Good carbs, bad carbs : an indispensable guide to eating the right carbs for
losing weight and optimum health / Johanna Burani and Linda Rao.
p. cm.
ISBN 1-56924-537-1
1. Reducing diets. 2. Glycemic index. 3. Carbohydrates in human nutrition.
I. Rao, Linda. M.Ed. II. Title
RM222.2 .B876 2002
613.2'5—dc21   2001055845

9 8 7 6 5 4 3

Designed by Pauline Neuwirth, Neuwirth & Associates, Inc.

Printed in the United States of America
DISTRIBUTED BY PUBLISHERS GROUP WEST

To Sergio, for teaching me about
selflessness and patience;

To Matteo, for teaching me about
trust and conviction;

To Paul, for teaching me about
generosity and sincerity;

To Dad, for teaching me
about integrity and love;

And to Mom, my first and best teacher.
You all are the wind beneath my wings.

Thank you. (J.B.)

To Mom and Dad, the most wonderful
and supportive parents anyone could have.
I treasure you.

To Maud, my beloved and my best friend. (L.R.)

> **Let thy food be thy medicine.**
>
> —Hippocrates

CONTENTS

PREFACE

When we started writing this book, our first task was to define our audience. Our goal was to provide readers unfamiliar with carbohydrates with an easy-to-understand introduction to these nutritional wonders—how they work, what they do, and why they're the most important type of food you can eat for good health and more energy. That's why you'll notice that this book is written in a conversational style, even though we do cover some technical topics.

Before we start talking about what this book includes, though, we'd like to be clear about what it *doesn't*: *Good Carbs, Bad Carbs* is neither a carbohydrate nor a physiology textbook, nor is it meant to be the definitive book on carbs. But if you've heard about carbs before and want to learn more about how they can benefit you, this book is for *you*!

Having said that, let's get the ball rolling by saying that in spite of the title *Good Carbs, Bad Carbs*, there are no bad carbs. Carbohydrates are important because your system selectively chooses them as its fuel of choice. And eating the *right* carbs—the slowly digested kind—can help you control blood-sugar levels, give you enough energy to sustain you throughout the day, help you lose weight easily and healthfully, and boost your heart health, as well. This book is about those carbs.

A Book in Two Parts

As you scan the contents, you'll see that the book is divided into two parts. In Part 1 we describe what carbs are: how they work and how your well-being and good health are affected by the amount and type of carbohydrates you eat.

Part 2 describes how eating slowly digested carbs can impact on weight loss, diabetes, and heart health. We aren't suggesting that eating carbohydrates *alone* can prevent diseases; no food by itself can do that. Our goal is only to point out that eating the *right kind* of carbs can positively influence many diseases. In addition, Part 2 also gives you the heads up on carb intake as it relates to kids and sports nutrition.

Now, after reading that Part 2 covers how carbs influence certain diseases, you might be tempted to start reading the book there. But we suggest that you start with Part 1 instead, because the information there lays the foundation for what you'll read later on. If you start at the beginning, you'll better understand the terms we use throughout this book and exactly why carbs work to positively affect your health.

Why You Need This Book

If you think that you're already pretty healthy—you don't have diabetes or heart disease or need to lose weight—you may wonder whether you need to read this book. Well, ask yourself these questions: Do you feel an energy dip midafternoon? Do you ever need to raid the fridge between meals because you feel hungry? Do you think that you could be eating better? If you answered yes to any of these questions, then this book may help you. And if you already suffer from overweight, diabetes, or heart disease, we'll show you how you can better manage your condition, reduce your risk of further complications, and feel much better too!

To your good health.

Johanna Burani, M.S., R.D., C.D.E.
Linda Rao, M.Ed.

PART 1

Carbohydrates: Your Body's Fuel of Choice

1

A BALANCED DIET DEFINED

Even though advertisements may claim otherwise, no one food will protect you from poor health. And as unhealthful as some foods may be, no one food will kill you. In fact, there are no bad foods—just bad diets. There are also good diets. How can you recognize the difference? And what is a diet anyway?

Diets vs. Diet

We've all heard so much about weight-loss diets; they may be called low-fat, or high-protein, or low-calorie diets, but they all aim to help you slim down. You may even have tried a few of these weight-loss plans in the past. If you have, you're not alone: Over the course of a given year, more than half of Americans either go on some type of weight-loss diet or try to maintain their weight. Unfortunately, few of them succeed at keeping the weight off.

And weight-loss diets aren't the only plans getting attention: You've probably also heard about high-fiber diets, and heart-healthful diets, and low-sodium diets. Though these programs aren't necessarily aimed at helping you to lose weight, they may, as a fringe benefit, do just that. So what, exactly, is a diet? Is it about losing weight, or what?

What Does "Diet" Mean?

The tenth edition of *Merriam Webster's Collegiate Dictionary* defines the noun *diet* as "food and drink regularly provided or consumed."

(By the way, some dictionaries also provide a second definition of *diet*: "to restrict oneself to special food, esp. in order to control one's weight; to feed esp. on special food as treatment or punishment." While dieting—by this definition anyway—can certainly feel like punishment, it isn't a nutritionist's working definition!)

So that's it . . . **a diet is how we normally eat.** This book explains how, with the right foods, your normal, everyday diet can help you achieve and maintain good health by providing you with a clear understanding of why carbohydrates are the single most influential nutrient in your diet—a diet that affects your day-to-day living, as well as your general health.

The 40-Plus Diet
(a.k.a. A Balanced Diet)

Let's start with the idea of a *balanced diet*. A balanced diet supports your good health by supplying you with the 40-Plus nutrients that you need every day. It consists of a wide variety and ample amount of nutrient-dense, healthful foods. (Nutrient-dense foods, by the way, are those foods that offer a lot of the good things your system needs—such as calcium, fiber, and protein, for example—for the calories it receives.) A balanced diet contains carbohydrates, protein, fat, vitamins, minerals, and water. While each of these nutrients functions as a team player, carbohydrate foods play the role of team captain.

Keeping all of these nutrients in mind when you're selecting foods from a restaurant menu or a supermarket shelf may seem like a tall order. It becomes easier, even *habitual*, though, when you focus on your health, at least most of the time. To help you,

Components of a Healthful Diet

Nutrient	Purpose	Food sources
TEAM CAPTAIN Carbohydrates	Serve as your body's primary energy source	Cereals, grains (including pasta, rice, barley, potatoes, and corn), legumes, fruits, vegetables, milk, and milk products
THE TEAM PLAYERS Fats	Serve as the stored-energy form that your system draws from when there aren't enough carbs	Red meat, fish, poultry, egg yolks, cheese (except non-fat), milk products (except non-fat), butter, margarine, oils, regular cream cheese and salad dressings, mayonnaise (except non-fat), seeds, and nuts
Proteins	Provide building blocks for organs, tissues, skin, bones, enzymes, and hormones	Red meat, fish, poultry, egg whites, cheese, tofu, milk and milk products, legumes, and nuts
Vitamins	Help your body develop and function normally; may guard against disease	Grains, fruits, vegetables, dairy products, meats, oils, nuts, and seeds
Minerals	Help your body develop and function normally; may guard against disease	Grains, fruits, vegetables, dairy products, meats, oils, nuts, and seeds
Water	Needed for all metabolic activities; helps transport glucose and other vital nutrients to cells; helps eliminate cellular waste products; helps you maintain a constant body temperature	Liquids such as water, juice, milk, soda, non-caffeinated beverages; to a lesser extent, water is in virtually all foods

the U.S. Department of Agriculture (USDA) and Health and Human Services (HHS) have published *Dietary Guidelines for Americans* to help all Americans focus on making healthful dietary and lifestyle choices. Updated every five years to reflect the most current information, the fifth edition of these guidelines was published in 2000.

Dietary Guidelines for Americans

Need help making healthful lifestyle choices? Here's some help, courtesy of the United States government:

- Aim for a healthy weight.
- Be physically active each day.
- Let the Food Guide Pyramid guide your food choices.
- Eat a variety of grains daily, especially whole grains.
- Eat a variety of fruits and vegetables daily.
- Keep food safe to eat.
- Choose a diet that is low in saturated fat and cholesterol and moderate in total fat.
- Choose beverages and foods that limit your intake of sugars.
- Choose and prepare foods with less salt.
- If you drink alcoholic beverages, do so in moderation.

From: *Dietary Guidelines for Americans,* fifth edition

These recommendations certainly provide us with a blueprint for healthful living that, based on current medical knowledge and research information, should support good, even optimal health. The third recommendation, "Let the Pyramid guide your food choices," calls our attention to the Food Guide Pyramid, another informational tool presented by the USDA and HHS to help all of us learn more about healthful eating.

Diagram of the Food Guide Pyramid

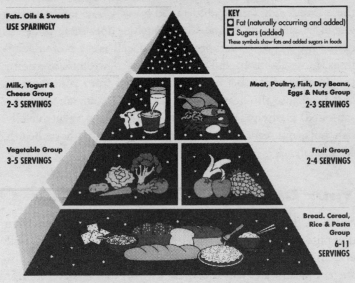

Fats. Oils & Sweets
USE SPARINGLY

KEY
▢ Fat (naturally occurring and added)
☑ Sugars (added)
These symbols show fats and added sugars in foods

Milk, Yogurt &
Cheese Group
2-3 SERVINGS

Meat, Poultry, Fish, Dry Beans,
Eggs & Nuts Group
2-3 SERVINGS

Vegetable Group
3-5 SERVINGS

Fruit Group
2-4 SERVINGS

Bread. Cereal,
Rice & Pasta
Group
6-11
SERVINGS

Source: United States Department of Agriculture and United States Department of Health and Human Services

You can see how the Food Pyramid goes hand in hand with the food recommendations of the *Dietary Guidelines.* Both of these tools stress the importance of eating balanced meals that contain lots of nutrient-dense foods and making daily food choices that include a wide variety of foods and moderate portion sizes. Both tools are designed to help you make eating a healthful *diet* a healthful *habit.*

The Food Guide Pyramid clearly stresses the importance of selecting foods from all the food groups. And while you need all groups for the best possible health, the Pyramid shows that the foundation of a healthful diet should come from grains (especially whole-grain breads and cereals, rice, and pasta, as you'll see emphasized throughout this book). The Pyramid also shows that you should be eating several servings of fruits and vegetables every day; in fact, some nutritionists recommend that 75 percent of your daily food servings should come from these three high-carbohydrate food groups. The fact is, eating lots of whole grains, fruits, and vegetables does seem to be the easiest way to get the carbohydrates, as well as the protein, vitamins, minerals, fiber, and water, you need without overdoing the amount of fat. Because you need fats from your diet, it's best to choose the heart-healthful kinds (mono- and polyunsaturated) as often as possible from foods such as vegetable oils, fish, nuts, and seeds. For more on dietary fats and heart health, see Chapter 7.

Your Diet: The Role Carbs Play

So all of this interest in grains, fruits, and vegetables in your diet puts these and other high-carbohydrate foods such as milk and milk products front and center on the good-nutrition stage. But how and why did these carbs get all this attention in the first place? If most of your food selections should come from these food groups, it's important to understand what your system gets from carbs.

First of all, let's repeat: You need protein, fat, vitamins, minerals, and water as well as carbohydrates to be healthy, and many foods offer an abundance of these vital nutrients. All of these nutrients play an important role in a well-balanced diet, and you should get them from high-carbohydrate foods (remember the Pyramid?). So why are carbs so critical? *Because they are your body's fuel of choice.*

Your system prefers to get its energy from the carbohydrates you eat rather than from either proteins or fats. Without going into the chemical explanation of why carbs get this special treatment (that comes later), for now, let's just say that your body recognizes that carbohydrates contain the greatest potential for providing energy. Somehow, your system knows that it's going to wind up with more glucose flowing in the bloodstream after you eat carbs than it will after you eat either proteins or fats. And your system wants to get as much energy as it can with the least amount of work.

So what do you get when you eat high-carbohydrate foods? Most of the energy you need for all your daily activities.

Carb Food Sources

High-carbohydrate foods include cereals, grains, legumes (such as lentils and kidney beans), fruits, vegetables, and milk products. Not coincidentally, most of these foods make up the bottom layers of the Food Guide Pyramid.

Your Diet: The Role Fat Plays

When it comes to getting quick energy from food, your system almost ignores dietary fats, although they do make an important contribution by providing you with the form of energy you can easily store to use later. Here's how fat storage works: Of all the nutrients you eat, fats contain the most calories. And because of the chemical structure of these calories, your body chooses them as its favorite nutrient for body-fat storage. You see, your system has been programmed, throughout evolution, to store *dietary* fats as *body* fat, to use in a possible future famine. Because most of us don't usually go hungry for more than a few hours at a time (or at all), we don't usually have a chance to dip into this stored fat for energy. Instead, you already know where it all goes: on your thighs, around your middle, and on your butt!

So, from fats, your body gets its best energy reserves. In fact, your system just loves to store fat and has an almost unlimited capacity to do so. The more fat stores it has, the happier it is. Not great news, is it? But this storage capacity explains, though, why it's such a good idea to cut back on fats if you're trying to lose weight.

Food Sources

Sources of dietary fats include red meat, fish, poultry, egg yolks, cheese (except non-fat), milk and milk products (except non-fat), butter, margarine, and oils, regular cream cheese and salad dressings, mayonnaise (except non-fat), seeds, and nuts.

Your Diet: The Role Protein Plays

Dietary proteins have a privileged status in your body: Protein foods provide the only building blocks your body uses to restore and repair itself. If your body were forced to use protein for energy because there weren't enough available carbs—its preferred fuel—it could; and it does, in extreme cases, such as during prolonged starvation. But breaking down protein for energy is a more complicated process and not one that your body easily performs.

So, from protein foods, your body gets the building units to make and maintain your organs, muscles, skin, tissues, and your entire lean body mass. Protein is vital for a healthy body, but watch out: Eat too many protein calories and your body won't make stronger or bigger muscles out of them—it will make body fat.

Protein Food Sources

The main protein sources include red meat, fish, poultry, egg whites, cheese, tofu, milk and milk products, as well as legumes and nuts.

So, at the end of the day, just what do you get from eating a well-balanced diet?

▶ Balanced proportions of carbohydrate (55 to 60 percent), protein (10 to 15 percent) and fat (less than 30 percent)

- Enough calories to meet your energy needs for the day
- At least the minimum amounts of most, if not all, of the 40-plus nutrients you need for good health

That doesn't sound so hard to do, does it? And eating this way makes you feel and look great!

THE BOTTOM LINE

➤ A diet is how we normally eat.

➤ A balanced diet supports good health by supplying you with the 40-plus nutrients that you need every day.

➤ Carbohydrates are your body's fuel of choice.

➤ Carbs give you the energy you need for all of your daily activities.

So-Sweet Pepper Soup

WHO would have thought that this humble combination of vegetables would produce such a hardy-tasting soup?

《 **Makes 9 cups   Serving size: 1 cup** 》

1 tbs.	olive oil
1	medium onion, coarsely chopped
1½	large celery stalks, coarsely chopped
2 cloves	garlic, minced
4 cups	low-sodium vegetable stock
2 cups	water
1½ cup (8 oz.)	creamer potatoes,* cubed
5	yellow bell peppers, halved, seeded, and quartered
½ tsp.	salt
⅛ tsp.	freshly ground pepper
3 cups	boiling water
1 cup	barley, uncooked

Homemade or commercial pesto sauce, to garnish (optional)

Grated reggiano Parmesan cheese, to garnish (optional)

1. In a large, wide-based saucepan, heat oil over medium-low heat. Add onions and celery; sauté 4 minutes. Add garlic and continue to sauté another 3 minutes (onions will be soft and translucent).
2. Add the next six ingredients (vegetable stock through ground pepper); bring to a boil. Reduce heat, cover and simmer for 40 to 45 minutes.
3. While the vegetables are cooking, in a separate medium saucepan bring 3 cups of water to a boil and add barley.
4. Reduce heat, cover, and simmer for 30 minutes; add more water if needed. Stir occasionally.
5. When cooked, drain barley and reserve in a large saucepan.

6. When vegetables are cooked, pour half of the mixture into a blender and process until completely smooth. Pour pureed mixture into pan with barley. Heat on low to keep warm.
7. Repeat with remaining pepper mixture. Stir thoroughly.
8. Garnish with nail-size dollop of pesto and grated cheese if desired.

> **EACH SERVING CONTAINS:**
> 116 calories, 24 grams carbohydrate, 3 grams protein, 2 grams fat, 0 milligrams cholesterol, 4 grams fiber

G.I.** = LOW
* Creamer potatoes are whole new potatoes with a thin, yellowish skin.
** Glycemic Index—See p. 150 for explanation.

2

How Carbs Work

Carbs, because they serve such an important function in your body, do require some explanation. And though we've done our best to simplify some very technical information, we know that for some people, this chapter won't exactly be a page-turner. But the concepts as we present them are relatively easy to understand, so hang in there. Because once you have a basic understanding of the facts in this chapter, you'll be able to better appreciate why carbs are the most important nutrient for everyday life. Ready? Let's go!

All of your body's functions, from breathing to moving to thinking, come from the energy molecules produce within your cells. And you get those molecules from the foods you eat. That's why food has a direct bearing on how well your body's energy works. But what are these molecules? What do they look like? What do they do?

Molecules Made Simple

Molecules are just tiny units from which everything around us is made—dogs and cats, sunflowers and bees, and the foods we eat. Your body is also composed of trillions of molecules. So what makes up a carbohydrate molecule? When you think of how many thousands, tens of thousands, of different carbohydrate-containing foods there are (including potatoes, chocolate chip cookies, apples and grapes, milk shakes, and fettuccine alfredo) it's almost shocking to learn that they all contain just three basic units, called atoms: carbon (C), oxygen (O), and hydrogen (H). In fact, that's how carbs get their name:

carbo = carbon (C)

hydrate = with water (H_2O)

These atoms join together (or bond) to form carbohydrate molecules. The different sizes and shapes of these carbohydrate molecules give special characteristics to the foods they're in. For example, carbohydrates in bread have a different chemical structure and size than carbohydrates in peaches—and that's why bread and peaches taste differently to us. But because these molecules are made of carbon, oxygen, and hydrogen, they are carbohydrates.

The Simple Carbohydrates

Simple carbohydrates are all sugars and fall into two categories: 1) one-molecule, or single sugars, or 2) two-molecule, or double sugars. The scientific names for these sugars are monosaccharides and disaccharides respectively. The most important monosaccharides are *glucose, fructose,* and *galactose.* The most important disaccharides are *maltose, sucrose,* and *lactose.* Your body breaks these double sugars down into at least one molecule of glucose and another single sugar.

In fact, this book is all about glucose: where it comes from in your diet and how you get it from the food you eat, what your system does with it, and why it prefers to use carbohydrates to get it.

The Monosaccharides: Glucose

Glucose, your body's "gasoline," is the most important of all the sugars in your system. It's the form of sugar that flows through your blood to provide energy to your cells and also serves as the structural unit of glycogen, one of your body's stored energy forms.

As a sugar, glucose tastes mildly sweet and occurs naturally in foods such as fruit and honey. In your body, it's hard to exaggerate glucose's importance: No other substance is more essential. Glucose is the form of energy that travels into your cells, allowing them to do their individual jobs. Every activity that every body cell performs occurs because of glucose. No glucose, no life. Now, *that's* how important it is!

What Do these Things Mean?

Troubled by some of the technical terms you see? Don't worry. Here's how those complex words break down into simple meanings:

mono = one

di = two

poly = many

saccharide = sugar

ose = sugar in

The Monosaccharides: Fructose

Fructose, also known as fruit sugar, is naturally found in all fruits, honey, and tree saps. It's the sweetest-tasting of all the naturally occurring sugars; you'll find it as an ingredient in some jellies, ice cream, cookies, yogurt, and other sweets. With a little help from your liver, fructose can be converted into the all-important energizer, glucose, or it can be stored as the starch, glycogen. And, if your glycogen stores are all filled up, you can also store fructose as fat.

What Is High-Fructose Corn Syrup?

This popular food ingredient is an intensely sweet sugar that food companies use to manufacture certain sweetened beverages, baked and frozen desserts, and some preserved foods, such as relishes and maraschino cherries.

The Monosaccharides: Galactose

This sugar helps to form the disaccharide lactose, which is important because lactose is the sugar contained in milk, an essential part of a balanced diet. Galactose is also a component of several bulking agents and stabilizers, such as carrageenan and guar gum, which are commonly used in many commercially prepared dessert and confectionery products.

Single sugars (Monosaccharides)

	Purpose	*Found in*
Glucose	Your body's number-one source of immediate energy; any excess will be stored as glycogen	Fruit, honey, sugar
Fructose	Used for immediate and stored energy	Fruit, honey, tree sap, sugar
Galactose	Used for immediate and stored energy	Milk and milk products, bulking agents used in chewing gum and ice cream

The Disaccharides: Maltose

Maltose, also called malt sugar, isn't used very often as a food ingredient. But here are two important things to know about maltose: First, it's a disaccharide, which means it's made of two simple sugars—in this case two glucose molecules. More simply put, your body takes one molecule of maltose and makes two glucose molecules out of it. Second, anytime you digest starch, your body breaks down the starch into maltose, which then breaks down into glucose. So on any given day, if you're eating a balanced diet as prescribed by the Food Guide Pyramid, you're taking in quite a few starch molecules. Your body easily digests 100 percent of these molecules into the sugar it's searching for—glucose.

White Bread's Tale

Have you ever let a piece of sliced white bread linger in your mouth long enough for the enzymes there to start digestion? If you did, you'd soon realize that the bread was starting to taste sweet, not starchy. What makes it sweet? The bread starch begins to break down into smaller and smaller molecules until the sugar (maltose) forms—and what's in every maltose molecule but two glucose molecules. That's where the sweetness comes from. Try it sometime!

The Disaccharides: Sucrose

Sucrose is the fancy name we give to table sugar. It's the sugar you put in your tea or coffee or sprinkle on your bowl of breakfast cereal. It's probably the sugar you're most familiar with; you may use it in baking and cooking, and you eat and drink it in some of the commercially prepared foods you eat throughout the day. Sucrose also occurs naturally in some plant juices or saps (such as maple syrup).

Here's why sucrose is so important: First, this disaccharide is made up of glucose and fructose. What does your body do with each sugar part? You can probably guess: It uses the glucose for immediate energy, and sends the fructose to the liver either to be converted into glucose for more immediate energy (if it's needed right then) or, more likely, the fructose goes into storage as glycogen so you can use it later on. This means that about half of the sucrose you eat becomes readily available energy, glucose.

When you compare the digestion of sugar to the digestion of a starch such as bread, you come to an astonishing conclusion: You get more quick energy from the *starch* in foods than you do from the *sugar* in foods. Why? Because starch breaks down into maltose, 100 percent of which becomes glucose, but only 50 percent of sucrose gets converted into glucose. Hold that thought for a little later on when we discuss how different kinds of carbs—both starches and sugars—affect blood-sugar levels and your health in general.

✔ **Food Fact**: According to the USDA's Human Nutrition Research Center statistics, Americans are currently consuming an average of 20 teaspoons of added sugar a day. That comes to about 300 calories!

✔ **Food Fact:** The USDA recommends consuming no more than *10 teaspoons of added sugar per day.* Ten teaspoons of sugar is exactly what's in *one 12-oz. can* of Dr Pepper or Pepsi, or *five* Starburst Fruit Chews.

Table Sugar 101

What is table sugar made from? Sucrose is actually refined sugar cane or sugar-beet juice that gets processed into granules (granulated sugar).

The Disaccharides: Lactose

Lactose, the sugar found in milk, is also a disaccharide; the simple sugars contained in it are glucose and galactose. The glucose part of lactose provides you with an immediate energy source, while the liver handles the galactose (much as it does with the fructose in sucrose). Lactose gives some people stomach trouble: Lactose-intolerant people have lower levels of the enzyme that breaks down this sugar in their intestines. When lactose sits in the gut and is poorly digested, it ferments, creating cramps, bloating, gas, and diarrhea. If this annoying and uncomfortable problem affects you, you may want to consume: 1) only small amounts of the offending foods, 2) lactose-reduced or lactose-free milk products, or 3) lactase capsules when you eat dairy foods.

> ✔ **Food Fact:** Lactose intolerance is not the same as a milk allergy, which is caused by a person's immune reaction to the protein in milk.

Double sugars (Disaccharides)

	Breaks down into	Purpose	Found in
Maltose	*glucose + glucose*	Used for immediate energy	Any starchy food
Sucrose	*glucose* + fructose	Used for immediate and stored energy	Table sugar
Lactose	*glucose* + galactose	Used for immediate and stored energy	All forms of milk and milk products

The Complex Carbohydrates

Some carbs are complex because they're much larger molecules than the simple carbs; they consist of many glucose units attached together, known chemically as a *polysaccharide*. The complex carbs consist of *glycogen* (how animals—including humans—store unused glucose), *starch* (how plants store unused glucose), and the *fibers* found in plant foods. Your body's digestive enzymes can't break down plant fibers; these fibers help form the bulk in your diet. Animals use their glycogen stores when the glucose supply is low; plants do the same thing with their starch reserves.

The Polysaccharides: Glycogen

Here's everything you need to know about glycogen: It's a complex carbohydrate found in your body but *not* in the food you digest. So where does it come from? Remember all those fructose and galactose molecules going to the liver? Well, the first thing the liver does with these molecules is to store them in a form that you can use later for quick energy (that is to say, a carb form rather than a fat form, which is the other form of stored energy we all know so well).

By the way, your liver also gives unused glucose molecules this same treatment: It also stores glucose as glycogen, which is made and stored in both the liver and muscle cells. Your body can use your liver's glycogen for immediate energy if it's needed to supplement a low glucose supply, such as during the night; but the muscles' glycogen usually sticks around to be used within the muscle cells. Because glycogen is made up of many glucose molecules, when you need energy from either your liver or your muscles, the molecules easily break apart the bonds holding the glucoses together. The result? A surge of energy—just what your body was looking for. Here we are, back to glucose again! And we're back to your body's retrieving glucose from its favorite fuel source, carbohydrates (in this particular case, glycogen).

The Polysaccharides: Plant Starch

Starch is to plants what glycogen is to humans: glucose in stored form. There can be hundreds, even thousands, of glucose molecules linked together to form a starch molecule, so they really are "big guys" in the molecule world. Plants such as yams or grains of rice store their energy—their glucose—as starch to use as needed for growth.

Luckily for us humans, we can digest most plant starches. Just think of all the times you've eaten wheat, corn, rice, and potatoes. There are lots of starches in our food supply, and your body knows how to break them down to get the fuel it needs—glucose.

✔ **Food Fact:** A 1-inch cube of a starchy food such as potatoes may contain as many as one million starch molecules.

The Polysaccharides: Plant Fibers

The fibers in plants are essential to their survival. These fibers support the plant and transport oxygen, water, and nutrients to all of its parts. We get dietary plant fibers from every plant we eat, whether it's a fruit or a vegetable, a grain or a legume, as long as the fibers haven't been removed during some refining process.

Like the other complex carbohydrates glycogen and starch, plant fibers are also polysaccharides; that is, they're also made up of many sugar molecules linked together. But there's a difference between the other polysaccharides and plant starches: Your body can't digest them at all. (To tell the truth, some fibers *can* be digested by some of the *bacteria* that live in the human gut but not by your body itself.) For this reason, plant fibers are defined as non-starch polysaccharides, or "unavailable" carbohydrates. (In contrast, all sugars, as well as glycogen and starch, represent your body's available sources of carbohydrates.) But don't think unkindly of fibers, because they still play an important role. Simply because they remain virtually intact in the gut, they help to lower blood cholesterol and slow down food digestion and glucose absorption (which is good for you, as we'll explain later). They also increase the bulk in your stool.

There are about seven different types of fibers important in your diet, and a few of them may even sound familiar: You may have come across these polysaccharides while following a high-fiber or weight-loss diet. You may also have seen fiber listed as an ingredient on many food labels.

Soluble Fiber

Four of the fibers are *soluble*: *pectins, gums, mucilages,* and some *hemicelluloses*. Your body's intestinal bacteria can digest these fibers, and as they do, the fibers break down into a gel. This gel does a host of wonderful things, such as lower cholesterol and regulate blood glucose levels for long periods of time. You'll find soluble fibers in plant foods such as oat and rice brans, rolled oats, barley, beans, carrots, and unpeeled apples, among others.

Where's the Fiber?

True or False? Foods derived from animal sources (meats, eggs, cheese, and milk, for example) contain no fiber.

Answer: True.

Insoluble Fiber

There are three types of *insoluble* fibers: *cellulose*, many *hemicelluloses*, and *lignans*. These fibers can absorb large amounts of water in the digestive tract, so they make up the bulk that you eventually eliminate. Here are some of the great things insoluble fibers do for you. They:

- decrease appetite
- slow the rate that your blood takes in the glucose that's formed from digested sugars and starches
- improve, or even cure, constipation
- decrease your risk of hemorrhoids, diverticulosis, and irritable bowel syndrome

Wheat bran (found in whole-grain cereals, breads, and crackers) is the richest source of insoluble dietary fiber. Other sources include legumes such as kidney, pinto, and lima beans.

Even though most of the fibers you eat don't produce glucose, they still affect how fast glucose gets dumped into your bloodstream. So even these carbs play an influential role in our day-to-day lives and overall good health. But there's still lots more to the story.

Complex Carbohydrates (Polysaccharides)

	Purpose	Found in
Glycogen	Used for quick-release from stored energy	No foods contain glycogen
Starch	Used for immediate energy	Wheat, corn, rice, potatoes
Plant Fibers	Decrease appetite	**Soluble:** oat and rice
	Slow the rate of glucose absorption	brans, rolled oats, barley, beans, carrots,
	Ease constipation	unpeeled apples
	Reduce risk of hemorrhoids, diverticulosis, and irritable bowel syndrome	**Insoluble:** wheat bran, legumes, fruits, vegetables

Why Are Carbohydrates So Important?

➤ Your body likes to get energy from carbohydrates; that's why carbs are your body's fuel of choice.

➤ Glucose is the energy form your body uses for all its activities.

➤ If you eat a balanced diet, at least half of your daily calories come from carbohydrates, so you're giving your body a majority of calories it will use for its energy needs, in the form it prefers.

Name That Sugar

Here are some common forms of sugar that you might find on a food's Nutrition Facts label:

➤ brown sugar

➤ cane sugar

> ➤ confectioners' sugar
> ➤ corn syrup
> ➤ crystallized cane sugar
> ➤ dextrin
> ➤ dextrose
> ➤ evaporated cane juice
> ➤ fruit juice concentrate
> ➤ high-fructose corn syrup
> ➤ honey
> ➤ invert sugar
> ➤ malt
> ➤ maltodextrin
> ➤ maple syrup
> ➤ molasses
> ➤ raw sugar
> ➤ turbinado sugar

Carbohydrate Digestion and Absorption

Question: Why does your body digest food?
Answer: To get the energy it needs to carry out all of its daily activities.

Question: What form of energy does your body use?
Answer: Glucose.

Question: Which are the easiest foods for your body to digest into glucose?
Answer: Carbohydrates.

Question: Why?
Answer: Because glucose is *already* a carbohydrate; your body doesn't have to work very hard to get energy from it. It likes that. That's why your body treats carbs preferentially.

Question: How does your body get the glucose and deliver it into the blood?

Answer: Keep reading!

Carb Digestion

To help illustrate the digestive process, let's follow the path of a piece of bread as it moves through your digestive system, starting with your mouth.

- With the help of your tongue, your teeth grind, tear, and pull the bread apart. Meanwhile, your saliva covers the bread.

- Amylase, a digestive enzyme in your saliva, begins breaking apart some of those huge starch molecules into shorter and shorter polysaccharides and eventually splits some of them into the disaccharide maltose. (Remember the experiment of holding a piece of bread in your mouth long enough to taste the sweetness of the maltose molecules?) This is a time-sensitive process, because food doesn't stay in your mouth for long.

- Once you swallow it, the bread travels down the esophagus and after a few minutes enters your stomach. The stomach works a little bit like a washing machine, bathing the bread in hydrochloric acid and gastric enzymes.

- When the "cycle" is finished, your stomach's acids have disinfected the bread. (And it's a good thing too: Consider all the bacteria you eat when you put food into your mouth.) In addition: 1) your body has digested the enzyme amylase that attached to the bread in your mouth, so its digestive role is over; 2) the hydrochloric acid splits whatever disaccharides have formed so far, mainly maltose into glucose; 3) more polysaccharides are breaking down into more disaccharides; and 4) any fibers in the bread have unraveled from the starch but remain undigested and linger in your stomach. This lingering slows down the movement of the just-formed simple carbohydrates into the small intestine.

▶ The next stop inside the digestive tract is the small intestine, a 20-plus-foot-long tube, the Grand Central Station of the whole digestive process. It's in the small intestine where most of the bread will be completely broken down.

▶ All of the starch molecules have by now become maltose molecules and then glucose molecules.

▶ The small intestine is the end of the line for just about all of the bread's digestion; any of the fiber in the bread will move down into the large intestine and be eliminated.

▶ The result of digestion: glucose; and possibly fructose and galactose if any ingredients, such as milk or sugar, have been added to the bread before baking.

Just as a reminder: We're describing carbohydrate digestion because this is a book about carbs. Your body also digests dietary proteins and fats, as we explained earlier.

Carb Absorption

To sum up: During digestion, your body breaks down carbs into the form of energy it can most immediately use, glucose, which is transferred from the intestinal cells into the blood. Your blood carries it throughout your body by *absorption*.

▶ Because of specialized cells on its lining, your small intestine is perfectly suited to transfer glucose out of the gut and into your bloodstream. These cells, called *villi*, look like tiny fingerlike projections.

- The villi allow glucose to leave the intestinal wall and get carried away by the circulating blood.
- The blood flows straight to and through the liver, where all of the monosaccharides (glucose and possibly fructose and galactose) are processed.
- The result of absorption: Glucose exits the liver and moves into the circulating blood and is ready for use.

So, to repeat:

Question: How does your body actually get the glucose from carbohydrate foods and deliver it into the blood? How does it use glucose as fuel?

Answer: It digests the food that has been eaten by passing it through the digestive organs (mouth, esophagus, stomach, small intestine, and liver) breaking it down further and further until it consists of just single sugars, which pass from the liver and into the bloodstream as glucose.

Glucose in Your Body and in Your Blood

Whew! That's a lot of work for your body to do, and it does the job every time you eat. But the job description isn't quite complete: What goes on once the glucose is finally circulating throughout your body? How do you extract energy from the glucose molecule?

First, the glucose molecule has to get *inside* the cell that needs the energy. We'll go into more detail about this process in a later chapter, but for now, the simple explanation is that a carrier (insulin) escorts the glucose into the cell.

- Once the glucose is inside the cell, many complicated chemical reactions have to occur in a certain sequence in order for it to produce the energy you need.

- Enzymes break the glucose molecule in half; these halves can be put back together again or they can be further broken down into smaller segments.
- Because the smaller segments can't be reassembled back into glucose, one of two things will happen to them: 1) they can be either turned into body fat; or 2) they can be completely broken down into three end products: carbon dioxide, water and . . . *energy.*
- As long as there's a constant supply of dietary carbs available, this process hums along with minimal effort. Remember, your body is well versed in turning carbs into energy.
- While you're digesting carbs into glucose for immediate energy, you're also digesting proteins into amino acids to meet your protein needs, and fats into fatty acids to store in your energy reserves. Insulin helps make all of these deliveries; its escort service allows your cells to receive the simplest digestive products: glucose, amino acids, and fatty acids.

So that is it, in a pretty big nutshell. The explanation above shows why carbohydrates are your body's fuel of choice and why your body wants to use carbs above all other nutrients for glucose, its energy source.

What's Insulin Anyway?

What is insulin?	It's a hormone.
Where is it made?	In your pancreas.
What does it do?	It controls the transport of glucose from the bloodstream into your cells.

Your Glycogen Stores

Your body collects a reserve of an easily broken-down starch supply called glycogen, which is stored in the liver and in muscle cells. The liver's glycogen stores add to the supply of energy to your brain, nerve cells, and other organs when your blood glucose levels are low. The muscles' glycogen stores (about twice the amount stored in the liver) are used by the muscles themselves. And remember: Your body dips into these supplies only when blood glucose levels are inadequate for its immediate energy needs.

THE BOTTOM LINE

➤ All living cells need glucose for energy.

➤ The six simple carbohydrates are glucose, fructose, and galactose, maltose, sucrose, and lactose.

➤ The three complex carbohydrates are glycogen, plant starch, and the plant fibers.

➤ Your body digests food by passing it through your digestive organs, breaking it down until it consists of simple sugars, amino acids, and fatty acids.

➤ Insulin escorts glucose, amino acids, and fatty acids into the cells where they're used.

Goat Cheese Wrap

HERE'S a quick grab-and-run sandwich. You can prepare it the night before and seal it tightly with plastic wrap. It'll still taste great the next day.

⟦ Makes 4 wraps   Serving size: 1 wrap ⟧

4 oz.	crumbled goat cheese
6	kalamata olives, coarsely chopped
¼ cup	marinated sun-dried tomatoes, thinly sliced
¼ cup	red onion, coarsely chopped
1 tsp.	olive oil
2 tsp.	balsamic vinegar
1 cup	arugula leaves, approx. 20
8	1-oz. slices low-salt boiled ham
4	2-oz. tortillas

1. Combine first 6 ingredients (goat cheese through vinegar) in medium bowl; set aside.
2. Chop arugula leaves, set aside.
3. Arrange 2 slices ham on each tortilla, overlapping them and placing them close to one end.
4. Spoon ¼ of cheese mixture on ham.
5. Top each tortilla with ¼ cup arugula leaves.
6. Starting at end with ham and cheese, completely roll up tortilla.
7. May be prepared and refrigerated several hours in advance.

EACH SERVING CONTAINS:
300 calories, 30 grams carbohydrate, 19 grams protein, 11 grams fat, 55 milligrams cholesterol, 2 grams fiber

G.I. = LOW

3

GUSHERS AND TRICKLERS:
AN INTRODUCTION

Let's recap what we've talked about so far: Your body ingests food, and in a balanced diet the majority of these food calories come from carbohydrates. Then your body digests this food for energy to do its daily work. The energy from these carbs takes a form called glucose; your body's preferred food source for glucose is carbohydrates.

Digesting food into glucose is a multi-step process, which, most of the time starts and finishes without your awareness that it's even going on. Once digestion is complete, the final products are properly packaged away: Amino acids (from protein digestion) head into cells so they can make more body protein or lean body mass; fatty acids (from fat digestion) move into cells as a form of stored energy; and the just-formed glucose molecules from carbohydrate digestion get packaged away too—into the bloodstream as the energy you will start using right away.

In order for glucose to be useful, though, it must get *inside* the cells. And, as we briefly mentioned in the last chapter, this is where that metabolic megastar, insulin, enters the picture. Here is how cells get "zapped" with energy:

> ● When glucose gets dumped into the bloodstream after digestion, it meets up with other glucose molecules already there. (The blood always contains some glucose.) Your brain starts a series of reactions that will eventually move the glucose out of your blood and into the cells, where it needs to be.

- Your brain activates the pancreas to secrete insulin. Why? Because the glucose can't move itself from the blood into the cells—it needs to be carried, and insulin is the carrier.

- Under normal conditions, the appropriate amount of insulin that your body needs for the actual sugar load at that time is the amount that your pancreas secretes into the blood.

- Now an insulin molecule picks up a glucose molecule and escorts it over to a cell. On the membrane of the cell there are several receptor sites; let's call them "doors." Insulin has the "key" to open the "door." Now the glucose molecule can enter the cell and give it the energy it needs to do the work it is supposed to do.

- As this process continues over time, more and more glucose gets moved into more and more cells and now you've got one pumped-up body that has the energy it needs to carry out its functions, day or night.

- After about four to five hours, your blood-sugar level starts to drop again, because for several hours, glucose has been moving out of your blood and into your cells nonstop. So, if we're awake, we eat, and the process starts all over again.

This summarizes what happens under normal circumstances in a healthy body, that is, a body without diabetes or glucose intolerance.

The Pancreas Profile

The pancreas is a soft grayish-white gland that rests behind the stomach and weighs just two or three ounces. It's about the size of a small, thick checkbook or a pencil case. This gland provides several of the enzymes you need to digest food into energy; it also makes hormones that help your body use that energy. The pancreas is the only place in your whole body that makes that ever-famous glucose-escort hormone, insulin. And it's only a certain kind of cell in the pancreas, the beta cell, that produces insulin. The special role that beta cells and the pancreas play makes them critical to good health: If, for some reason, the beta cells can't produce insulin, the glucose that has entered the blood after digestion has nowhere to go, so it stays in the blood. Too much glucose can lead to elevated blood sugars, which may result in diabetes.

> *Did You Know . . .* that your pancreas changes from grayish-white to a rosy pink when it's secreting insulin?

The Beta Business

Beta cells make and secrete insulin. In fact, these cells make insulin all the time, but if you haven't eaten, their activity is minimal. But once the food you eat enters your gut and digestion starts to elevate blood-glucose levels, the beta cells are stimulated to step up their insulin production. At first—a minute or two after you eat—stored insulin shoots out into the blood. In the meantime, the beta cells start working full force and continue to secrete insulin as it's needed. Usually the resting (or "basal") level of insulin secretion returns within three hours after you've eaten your meal or snack.

✔ **Fun Fact:** There are millions of beta cells in the pancreas.

> *Did You Know . . .* that a healthy pancreas secretes 20 to 30 units of insulin every day?

"Gushers" vs. "Tricklers"

How well your body functions at specific times depends on how quickly it makes glucose available to expectant cells—the difference between "gusher" foods and "trickler" foods. For example, sometimes you need a surge of energy (from a gusher) because the blood-sugar level is low; orange juice will do a better job of quickly raising the sugar level than an egg and cheese sandwich or a milk shake. At other times, you're looking for a steady stream of a more constant flow of energy (from a trickler), such as when you're taking a three-hour hike or wallpapering a room. Then, a bowl of rolled oats with milk and peaches will provide this kind of sustained energy better than a sleeve of salty crackers or some rice cakes with jelly. That's the difference between gushers and tricklers. (See the chart below for an illustration of how tricklers offer a steady release of energy compared to gushers.)

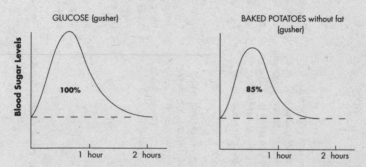

Adapted from *The Glucose Revolution Pocket Guide to Diabetes.* Reprinted courtesy of Marlowe & Company.

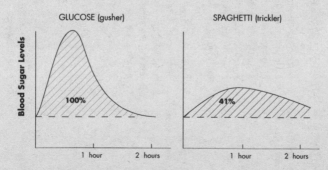

Adapted from *The Glucose Revolution.* Reprinted courtesy of Marlowe & Company.

	Gushers	Tricklers
What types of food?	Quickly digested carbohydrates	Slowly digested carbohydrates
Why are the foods digested this way?	Because of the major ingredient in a food (such as enriched wheat flour in white bread) or because of the extensive processing methods used to manufacture a food (like puffing up Rice Krispies or rice cakes), your body has a quick and easy time of breaking down the carb molecules into glucose, allowing for rapid digestion.	Because of the major ingredient in a food (such as 100% stoneground whole-wheat flour in whole-grain bread) or because of the minimal processing (such as in rolled oats rather than instant oats), your body has much more work to do to break the carb molecules into glucose; they will all be digested, but the process will take much longer to complete.
How does digestion happen?	Once the glucose molecules are readied in the small intestine, they exit into the blood. If many molecules are ready at the same time (or "gush") into the blood, they will all leave at the same time, creating a surge, or spike, of blood sugar.	If the starch molecules in, say, a slice of 100% whole-wheat bread are protected by several layers of fibrous tissue (bran), or if they are compressed into a tiny dense product such as Bran Buds, the digestive enzymes have a lot of breakdown work to do. It's as though the starch molecules are on a slow-moving conveyor belt going through the small intestine, where, at each station a little more, and then a little more, of the starch gets broken down. When a glucose molecule is finally produced, it hops off the conveyor belt and into the blood. This process produces a more constant, even flow (a "trickle") of energy for a longer period of time.
Examples	Cornflakes, sticky rice, rice cakes, dates, Gatorade, instant oatmeal	Bran, al dente pasta, yams, milk, rye bread, cookies, apples

The Roller-Coaster Effects of Gushers

In a glucose-tolerant, non-diabetic person, if blood sugars gush up because of eating many quickly digested carbohydrate calories, they're going to come crashing down. (Review: This is because your body meets the high sugar load with a huge outpouring of insulin from the pancreas and also because the cells are sensitive to insulin's presence and open up to let the glucose inside them.) So, as a result, first there's a lot of sugar in the blood, and then there's a lot less sugar in the blood, because now it has moved into the cells.

This rapid rise—then drop—in glucose levels can make you feel hungry, tired, shaky, headachy, unfocused, and irritable—the classic signs of low blood sugar (also called *hypoglycemia*). It's interesting to note that these are also the classic symptoms that many chronic dieters experience.

hypo = low
glyc = sugar
emia = blood

If you have type 2 diabetes, the most common form of the disease, gushers bring blood-sugar levels up, and then your body has a difficult time lowering those levels again. (Another review: This is due to insufficient insulin and/or the lack of cooperation from the cells to allow the glucose to enter them.)

If you don't have diabetes, a steady diet of gushers makes you hungry, tired, and irritable. If you do have diabetes, gushers make blood-sugar control more difficult. And here's another unfriendly effect that gushers can have—in people with or without diabetes: They encourage you to store fat—how unfriendly is that? Why would gushers lead to fat storage? Because gusher calories force more insulin to circulate in the blood, and the more insulin moving around in the blood, the greater the likeli-hood that some glucose will be put away into storage as fat.

Cruise Control with Tricklers

By their very definition, slowly digested carbs, or tricklers, don't give blood-sugar levels much of a roller-coaster ride—heck, they barely give them a carousel ride! Tricklers provide a more steady, even energy flow into the blood (as glucose molecules become available from the small intestine), and promote a more constant flow of energy out of the blood and into the cells. It's like driving a car in cruise control; with little effort, a steady, even flow of fuel passes through the motor and keeps the car running smoothly until it is time for another fill-up.

Your body performs as well as the car when its energy (or fuel) supply is constant: You have the right amount of energy to draw from for your daily activities, those you deliberately perform, such as climbing stairs or working at a computer, as well as those activities that you perform without realizing it, such as breathing and digesting your breakfast. With adequate energy, your body feels in control of its energy supply; it knows it won't run dry and can make it to the next fill-up. Better yet, by eating slowly digested carbs, you don't feel that tongue-hanging exhaustion at the end of the day. Slowly digested calo-ries from trickler foods at lunch provide you with a sense of fullness until you can prepare and eat dinner at night. This con-stant energy supply will not only keep you feeling satisfied from meal to meal, it will also help you to make better, controlled food choices—not impulsive ones that result from feeling rav-enously hungry, tired, and hypoglycemic.

As if these benefits of tricklers were not enough, there's another bonus to eating them: They discourage your body from storing glucose as fat by encouraging it to use the glucose for immediate energy. No fat stores piling up here! Now, that is really good news, isn't it? Eat a well-balanced diet, which includes "trickler" carbs in adequate, not excessive, amounts, and lose weight. (We'll talk more about the weight-loss advantages of trickler carbs later, in Chapter 5.)

The Gusher/Trickler Identification Profile

You can tell whether a food is a gusher or a trickler by. . .

▶ How much a starch swells up when it's cooked
    Gushers: A lot
        Examples: Sticky rice, overcooked pasta
    Tricklers: A little
        Examples: Long-grain rice, brown rice, *al dente* pasta
▶ How fibrous the food is
    Gushers: Low fiber content
        Examples: Bagels, hard rolls, cornflakes
    Tricklers: High fiber content
        Examples: Whole-grain breads, All-Bran, lentils, barley
▶ How much processing (pumping in air, refining, or milling of whole grains) the food has undergone
    Gushers: A lot
        Examples: Rice cakes, instant oatmeal, enriched wheat breads
    Tricklers: Minimal
        Examples: Old-fashioned or rolled oats, 100% whole-wheat bread
▶ How acidic the food is
    Gushers: Low acid content
        Examples: Chocolate cake and devil's food cake
    Tricklers: High acid content
        Examples: Sourdough bread products and buttermilk pancakes

> How sweet the food is
>> **Gushers:** A lot of sugar, with little or minimal fiber, protein, or fat
>>> **Examples:** Gatorade, sugar wafers
>> **Tricklers:** Some sugar, also containing some fiber, protein, or fat
>>> **Examples:** Social Tea biscuits, shortbread, arrowroot cookies

How to Calculate a Mixed Meal

Keep in mind that when eaten *alone,* gusher foods will cause their signature glucose spike and, when eaten *alone,* tricklers cause a longer-lasting supply of sugar in the blood. But what happens when we eat a meal that has a *mix* of gushers and tricklers? Well, first remember that the glucose is coming from the *carbohydrates* in your meal, so you want to look at only those—which types and how much of them you ate. Then you want to consider how much a part of the entire carb intake each carbohydrate food contributes (is it 10 percent of all the carbs in the meal, or 50 percent, or how much?). When you add it all up, if there are more gusher calories being digested from the meal, you'll experience a more rapid rise in blood sugar than if you had eaten more trickler calories. (The presence of proteins and fats in the meal will also influence glucose levels, but we'll talk more about that in the next chapter.)

THE BOTTOM LINE

▶ Gusher, or quickly digested foods, create blood-sugar spikes that leave you feeling hungry, tired, and irritable. They may encourage fat storage.

▶ Trickler, or slowly digested foods, keep your blood sugar on an even keel, so you feel energized and full. They discourage fat storage.

▶ How quickly your body digests a carbohydrate depends on its ingredients and its processing and preparation.

Spaghetti Estate

SURPRISE! Here's a refreshing salad that serves as a "sauce" for spaghetti. This recipe is adapted from a small trattoria in the heart of Rome, famous for its "Summer Spaghetti."

❴ **Makes approx. 10 cups, combined pasta and sauce (4 servings)** ❵
Serving size: Approx. 1 cup pasta; approx. 1⅓ cups sauce

4 qts.	water
1 tbs.	coarse salt
6 oz.	spaghetti (approx. ⅓ box)
1 lb.	tomatoes-on-the-vine, seeds removed and sliced into bite-sized pieces*
6 oz.	fresh mozzarella, cut into bite-sized cubes
20	fresh basil leaves, *hand-ripped* into small pieces
2 tbs.	olive oil
	salt to taste, optional

1. Bring 4 quarts water to a rolling boil in a large pot. Add salt.
2. Add spaghetti to boiling water. Stir until all strands are completely submerged.
3. Once water returns to a boil, cook pasta, uncovered, for 8 minutes, stirring occasionally. DO NOT OVER-COOK.
4. While pasta is cooking, prepare the tomatoes, mozzarella, and basil and place each in a separate small bowl.
5. When the pasta is cooked *al dente*, drain and return to pot. Toss with olive oil. Cool slightly.
6. Divide pasta equally into four bowls.
7. For the uncooked sauce: In each of the individual bowls on top of the pasta, prepare 3 concentric circles

starting at the outer rim. In the outermost circle, form a large border of cut tomatoes. Then form a circle of the cheese cubes. In the center, place a small mound of basil. Sprinkle salt over sauce, if desired. Serve immediately.

> **EACH SERVING CONTAINS:**
> 364 calories, 38 grams carbohydrate, 15 grams protein, 17 grams fat, 33 milligrams cholesterol, 2 grams fiber

G.I. = LOW

*Tomatoes should be ripe but firm.

4

THE GLYCEMIC INDEX:
A WAY TO RANK CARBS

Why is it that we know so much about gushers and trick-lers? After all, it's not like there are reporters inside the small intestine or the blood or the liver giving firsthand updates twenty-four hours a day, every day. The differing effects of quickly digested and slowly digested carbohydrates on blood-sugar levels are now common knowledge thanks to the unrelenting efforts of several researchers who understood what was happening in carbohydrate digestion and sought to prove it scientifically.

In 1981 scientists in Toronto were researching which foods were best for people with diabetes. Up to that time, people with diabetes were given dietary exchanges to follow, that is, certain foods in certain portions could be substituted or exchanged for other nutritionally similar foods. So, for example, a half cup of mashed potatoes could easily be "exchanged" in a meal for a half cup of pasta. The presumption was that these two starches would produce the same blood-sugar response once they were digested—and that the response would be a slow, modest rise of glucose into the blood. And the other piece of advice given to people with diabetes was that they should avoid sugar and not be too concerned about bread, rice, potatoes, and so on, since these were starchy (not sweet) carbs and, therefore, would not produce high rises in sugar levels.

When these ideas were actually put to the test in the Toronto labs, scientists made an astonishing discovery: The investigators found, for example, that fruits such as apples or grapes, despite their sugar content, caused blood sugars to rise less than plain sliced white bread! But how could that be? Weren't sugars supposed to raise blood sugar and weren't starches supposed to have less effect on blood sugars?

That wasn't what the researchers found: Their laboratory tests proved that some foods with sugar did not produce the expected high, rapid rise in blood-sugar levels, while some starchy foods did. In other words, the new dietary message for people with diabetes was that some starches elevate blood sugars as much as, or even more than, some sweet or sugary foods. This research gave birth to the Glycemic Index (G.I.), what we're informally calling gushers and tricklers.

The Glycemic Index is a ranking of carbohydrates based on their immediate effect on blood-sugar levels. All of the foods the researchers tested are compared with a reference food, such as pure glucose. (See illustration on page 35.) The ranking is based on a scale of 0 to 100. Glucose has a G.I. value of 100 because it doesn't have to break down any further. The more quickly a carbohydrate breaks down into glucose, the closer its G.I. value is to 100. And the more slowly a carb becomes glucose, the lower its G.I. value. Here we are—back to gushers and tricklers again!

The Research Continues

Scientists around the world continue to test carbohydrate foods for their Glycemic Index values. In fact, to date, researchers have tested more than 600 commonly eaten carbohydrates. Clinical studies throughout the world prove that the Glycemic Index is a valid tool for blood-sugar control. You can find more detailed information about the Glycemic Index on the following two Web sites:

- *www.glycemicindex.com*
- www.mendosa.com/gi.htm

Part 2 of this book illustrates specific health advantages of choosing low-G.I. foods over high-G.I. foods when you eat them as part of a balanced (mostly carb) diet. Some of those benefits include blood-sugar control, weight management, heart health, athletic performance, and endurance. But the best side effect from a low-G.I. diet is how good it makes you feel!

Did You Know . . . that "glycemic" means "sugar" + "in blood"?

The Glycemic Index: What's In, What's Out

Which foods will you find listed in the Glycemic Index?
Carbohydrates.
Which foods won't you find listed in the Glycemic Index?
Proteins and fats.

Brain Teaser #1:

Why are *only* carbohydrate foods listed in the Glycemic Index?

➤ Which foods are your body's fuel of choice?
Carbohydrates.

➤ In a balanced diet, which foods contribute the most calories to be used for energy? *Carbohydrates.*

➤ Which, of all the foods you eat, most affects blood-sugar levels? *Carbohydrates.*

➤ If the Glycemic Index focuses on those foods that most affect blood-sugar levels, which foods would it be looking at? *Carbohydrates.*

Now you know why carbs are the only foods listed in the Glycemic Index.

Brain Teaser #2:

High-protein foods and fats *aren't* listed in the Glycemic Index. Why not?

➤ Which, of all the foods you eat, most affects blood-sugar levels? *Carbohydrates.*

➤ Which, of all the foods you eat, least affects blood-sugar levels? *Proteins and fats.*

➤ Why don't protein foods affect blood-sugar levels? *Because the majority of protein calories are used to restore and rebuild the many different body cells; they're not normally converted into glucose for immediate energy.*

➤ Why don't fats affect blood-sugar levels? *Because your body puts 95 percent of fats into storage for future,* rather than *immediate,* energy use.

➤ What's the purpose of the Glycemic Index? *To rank those foods that affect blood-sugar levels.*

➤ Which foods most affect blood-sugar levels? *Carbohydrates.*

➤ Which foods does the Glycemic Index rank? *Carbohydrates.*

Now you know why high-protein foods and fats aren't listed in the Glycemic Index.

Note: Exceptions to the protein and fat rule include milk and yogurt, and legumes such as lentils and chickpeas. These foods are high in protein (and sometimes fat) but they also have a high carbohydrate content, which is why they've been tested and included in the Glycemic Index.

The Glycemic Index in a Typical Meal

Does the Glycemic Index apply to meals as it does to individual carbs? What happens when we eat a meal that contains many foods, including gushers and tricklers? Well, first keep in mind that your after-meal blood-sugar level is coming from the carbs you've eaten—which types and how much of them. And then, the presence of proteins, fats, fiber, and acidic foods will also influence how quickly glucose gets into your bloodstream. Can you imagine: Your body takes all of this into account before blood-sugar levels rise after a meal?

Rating the Glycemic Index of Foods

Food	G. I. Value
High G.I. (gusher)	greater than 70
Intermediate	55–70
Low G.I. (trickler)	less than 55

High-G.I. Foods

- Kellogg's Corn Flakes (84)
- General Mills' Cheerios (74)
- Rice cakes (82)
- Watermelon (72)
- Gatorade (78)
- Instant mashed potatoes (86)
- Baguette (95)

Intermediate-G.I. Foods

- Corn (55)
- Nabisco Social Tea biscuits (55)
- Ice cream (61)
- Quaker chewy granola bar (61)
- Pea soup (66)
- Long-grain white rice (56)
- Rye bread (65)

Low-G.I. Foods

- Skim milk (32)
- Orange (44)
- Macaroni (45)
- Strawberry jam (51)
- Whole-grain pumpernickel bread (51)
- Baked beans (48)
- Chickpeas (42)

So what's so great about the Glycemic Index? Simple—it illustrates how blood-sugar levels are affected by how quickly or how slowly you digest carbohydrates. The Glycemic Index spells it all out for you: Foods with a high Glycemic Index are gushers, while foods with a low Glycemic Index are tricklers. It's as simple as that! To make things even easier, in the appendix of this book, we've categorized a long list of carbohydrate foods into just three categories: trickler, intermediate, and gusher.

THE BOTTOM LINE

➤ Some starches elevate blood sugars as much as, or even more than, some sugary or sweet foods.

➤ The Glycemic Index ranks carbohydrates based on their immediate effect on blood-sugar levels.

➤ Tricklers are foods with a low Glycemic Index value.

➤ Gushers are foods with a high Glycemic Index value.

➤ Low-G.I. foods = slowly digested carbs = tricklers

Old World Vegetable Stew

THIS versatile mixture of vegetables and herbs will enhance the flavors of rice, pasta, couscous, or pita bread. It mixes so well with so many staples, it can easily become a staple itself!

❴ Makes 10 servings   Serving size: 1 cup ❵

2 tbs.	olive oil
1	large garlic clove, minced
2 medium	onions, thickly sliced
1 medium	eggplant (approx. 12 oz.), unpeeled and cubed
1 medium	sweet red pepper, seeded and sliced into 2-inch strips
1 medium	green bell pepper, seeded and sliced into 2-inch strips
2 large	yellow or green squash, thickly sliced
4 medium	tomatoes, peeled and seeded, cut into eighths (or 1 20-oz. can of plum tomatoes, drained, seeded, and quartered)
1 12-oz.	jar marinated artichoke hearts, drained and quartered
1 tbs.	fresh thyme (½ tsp. dried thyme)
1 tbs.	fresh oregano (½ tsp. dried oregano)
2 tbs.	fresh basil, minced, or 1 tsp. dried
⅛ cup	balsamic vinegar
½ tsp.	freshly ground black pepper
2 tbs.	fresh parsley, finely chopped

1. Heat oil in large saucepan. Add garlic and onions, and cook over low heat until onions are soft.
2. Add eggplant, peppers, and squash and continue to cook over medium heat for 5 minutes, stirring frequently.
3. Add tomatoes, artichoke hearts, and herbs and mix well. Cover and simmer for 20 minutes, stirring frequently.

4. Stir in the balsamic vinegar. Continue to cook, uncovered, for 5 minutes, stirring frequently.
5. Add black pepper and parsley; mix thoroughly. May be served hot or at room temperature.

EACH SERVING CONTAINS:
101 calories; 15 grams carbohydrate; 1 gram protein; 6 grams fat; 4 grams fiber, 0 milligrams cholesterol

G.I. = LOW

Good Carbs: Your Edge Against Disease

5

EAT GOOD CARBS,
LOSE WEIGHT

When it comes to talking about the obesity problem in
this country, you already know the story; in fact, many of us are
characters in the tale. But if we're overweight, it isn't for lack of
trying to be slimmer, that's for sure. You can't step into any
public place without hearing someone say that they're on a
"diet." In fact, do you know what percentage of U.S. adults are
"dieting?" Seventy-three percent. Yet for all the hunger pangs,
deprivation, calorie cutting, and family-room exercise equipment many of us live with, most weight-loss diets just don't
work over the long term. Take a look at these statistics:

- Six out of ten American adults (97 million people) are
  overweight or obese.
- One in four American children (ages 6 to 17) are overweight.
- In the past twenty years, the percentage of adult
  Americans who are grossly overweight or obese has
  nearly doubled to 26 percent. (Read: Not only are we
  gaining weight, we're gaining *a lot* of extra weight.)
- The cost to treat obesity-related health problems is
  estimated at approximately $100 *billion* a year.
- Obesity-related health problems are the second leading cause of death in America, accounting for about
  300,000 deaths a year.
- In 1994, more than 39 million lost workdays were
  related to obesity.

❭ More than 89 million sick-in-bed days were related to obesity in 1994.

❭ In 1994, more than 62 million doctor visits were related to obesity.

These numbers give us an idea of the extent of the problem. Now, what exactly *is* the problem? Who's considered overweight? Who's considered obese? Do *you* have some weight to lose?

Overweight or Obese or What?

Let's face it: You can tell whether or not you're carrying around extra weight. Maybe your clothes are getting too tight, maybe it just takes more effort to bend over to tie your shoes or maybe that bus or plane seat feels a little too snug. No matter what the sign, you don't need someone else—your doctor, your spouse, or your best friend—to tell you. No one knows better than you do. Sure, you could *think* that you're overweight and not be. That's also a medical problem, but not our focus right now. For most of us, if we think we're overweight, we probably are. But let's not be judgmental; let's go with the facts. First, let's define some terms so you know exactly what we're talking about.

> **Did You Know . . .** that obesity is the second leading cause of *preventable* death in the U.S.? (Only smoking kills more people.)

Determine Your Body Mass Index (BMI)

Measuring your BMI is the most popular way to determine whether you're overweight. This measurement shows the relationship of your weight to your height. Here's how you calculate BMI:

BMI =weight (lbs.) × 705 ÷ height (in.)²

Example: Let's say that you're 5'9" and weigh 250 pounds. Here's how you would calculate your BMI:

250 lbs. x 705 ÷ 69 in. x 69 in. = 176,250 ÷ 4,761 = 37 (BMI)

What Your BMI Means

So, now you know how to determine your BMI. But what does the number mean? Here are some guidelines:

Classifications	BMI
▶ Underweight	less than 18.5
▶ Normal weight	18.5–24.9
▶ Overweight	25–29.9
▶ Mild obesity	30–34.9
▶ Moderate obesity	35–39.9
▶ Extreme obesity	more than 40

Take a look at the BMI classifications above and fill in the blanks: "I'm _____ because my BMI is _____." For example: "I'm moderately obese because my BMI is 37."

What's a Healthy Weight?

You may have read or heard people talking about a "healthy" or "desirable" body weight. But what exactly do these words mean? You're at a healthy weight if you:

▶ meet standards of a weight guideline such as *Dietary Guidelines for Healthy Americans,* or the Body Mass Index chart.

- have the kind of body-fat distribution that lowers your risk of disease or death, which means that your body shape is more like a pear than an apple
- are at a weight that doesn't cause you to develop an unhealthy medical condition
- have a BMI of less than 25

Here are some examples of healthy weights:

- 5'10" man, 170 lbs.
- 5'5" woman, 130 lbs.
- 5'6" adolescent boy, 140 lbs.
- 5'1" teenage girl, 115 lbs.

Overweight: To be considered overweight, you must weigh no more than 10 percent above the desirable weight for your height. (Your BMI will measure between 25 and 29.9.) Research shows that if your BMI is greater than 28, you're at much greater risk for stroke, heart disease, and type 2 diabetes.

Here are some examples of overweight:

- 5'10" man, 190 lbs.
- 5'5" woman, 160 lbs.
- 5'6" adolescent boy, 180 lbs.
- 5'1" teenage girl, 140 lbs.

Obese: You are considered obese if your body weight is greater than 10 percent above the desirable weight for your height. (The BMI for an obese person will be 30 or more.) There are three classes or degrees of obesity:

Class 1 (mild)	BMI = 30–34.9
Class 2 (moderate)	BMI = 35–39.9
Class 3 (extreme)	BMI = 40 or higher

Here are some examples of obese weights:

- 5'10" man, 220 lbs. (mild); 250 lbs. (moderate); 300 lbs. (severe)
- 5'5" woman, 190 lbs. (mild); 220 lbs. (moderate); 260 lbs. (severe)
- 5'6" adolescent boy, 190 lbs. (mild); 230 lbs. (moderate); 250 lbs. (severe)
- 5'1" teenage girl, 160 lbs. (mild); 190 lbs. (moderate); 220 lbs. (severe)

Health professionals often use a person's BMI to help them determine if that person's weight is a risk factor for poor health. The only time the BMI might not accurately predict weight as a risk factor is when it's used to measure very muscular or athletic people, because their bodies will have a very high percentage of lean muscle mass. And because muscle weighs more than fat, the heavier weight could indicate a high BMI for that person's height. In a muscular person, though, a heavier weight may not be a disease risk factor at all. Just to be sure, there's another body measurement that you can take right in your own home: It's your waist circumference.

Waist Circumference

In addition to BMI, waist circumference (the distance around your waist) is important, because research shows that extra abdominal fat is a serious risk factor for such health concerns as type 2 diabetes, high blood pressure (hypertension), heart (cardiovascular) disease, and elevated cholesterol. The following waist measurements indicate excess abdominal fat, which would put you at greater disease risk:

Men   40 inches or more
Women   35 inches or more

(Read more about body shapes on page 99.)

What Causes Overweight and Obesity?

You know there's no escaping from the widespread, ever-present influences of living with super-sized, cheap, easy-to-find-any-time-of-the-day-or-night fast food, empty-calorie meals, and snacks. Bingo! That's actually the definition of many Americans' meals: the same people who are trying to "diet." There's also no escaping from the very real fact that we're not winning the weight war; we aren't even coming out ahead in a small battle once in awhile.

So our obesity statistics are climbing because we eat too many poor quality calories. But our collectively poor diet is not the only culprit for our national weight problem. What about our couch potato lifestyles and our sky-high levels of daily stress? Believe it or not, there was a time when, as Americans, life wasn't so hectic, when meals and mealtimes were actually given their importance throughout the day, three times a day. To illustrate the point, we've compared the typical schedules of Rose, a stay-at-home mom from the 1950s and Mary, the new millennium supermom. We think you'll agree: What a difference just fifty years can make!

Rose's Story

Rose was a happily married homemaker. She lived in a two-family house in an urban neighborhood, where her parents lived on the ground floor and she and her family above them. Her husband worked for a large furniture store in a big city. They had two teenage children; the son traveled forty-five minutes by train to his high school and the daughter walked to the local high school. Most stores were within walking distance. Rose had no major health problems, although some longstanding childhood illnesses had left her with mild anemia and some visual disability. In general, though, she lived the lifestyle of a strong, healthy forty-three-year-old woman. She was 5'1" tall and weighed 118 pounds, which comes out to a BMI of 22, a healthy weight. Here's what one of Rose's typical days looked like:

Morning

6:30: Woke up, prepared breakfast and lunches for the family

Breakfast: Orange juice, buttered toast, poached egg, cup coffee or glass whole milk

7:30–9:00: Sent family off to work or school; washed, dried, and put away breakfast dishes; swept kitchen floor; made beds; tidied up bathroom; put load of dirty laundry in washing machine (in the basement); got dressed in street clothes for daily marketing

9:00–11:00: Walked to the grocer, the butcher, and the bakery

11:00–11:15: Walked home, either carrying brown paper bundles or wheeling a pushcart depending on the number of items to carry

11:15–11:45: Delivered groceries to her mother and put away all bought items, went down to basement, unloaded washed laundry into basket, and hung clothes on outdoor laundry line

11:45–12:15: Prepared and ate lunch

Lunch: Ham and cheese sandwich on white bread with mustard, lettuce, and tomato, piece of fruit, water

Afternoon

12:15–12:30: Cleaned up after lunch and washed, dried, and put away dishes

12:30–1:30: Took a nap

1:30–3:00: Began prep work for dinner meal: Made salad; started homemade vegetable soup; cleaned whole chicken and prepared it for oven roasting; cut up roasting vegetables. Picked up dried laundry

3:00–3:15: Made snack for daughter arriving home from school, sprinkled water on laundry to be ironed

3:15–4:45: Put chicken roaster and vegetables in oven, ironed

4:45–5:00: Removed ironing board from kitchen, set dinner table, made final preparations for evening meal

Evening

5:15–5:30: Husband and son returned home, everyone washed up for dinner

5:30–6:15: Family ate dinner together

Dinner: Homemade vegetable barley soup, oven-roasted chicken, roasted potatoes and carrots, lettuce and tomato salad, homemade vinaigrette dressing, piece of fruit, water

6:15–6:45: Cleaned up, washed, dried, and put away dishes, folded and put away tablecloth and cloth napkins, swept floor

6:45–7:00: Made and served after-dinner dessert

Snack: Cup of coffee and coffee cake

7:00–9:00: Watched TV or read; mended if necessary

9:00–9:15: Washed up and went to bed

Keep in mind that in 1950, Rose had to do without these handy time- and energy-savers:

- Steam iron
- Remote control for the TV
- Clothes dryer
- Permanent press (no-iron) clothing
- One-stop megamarkets
- Food processor
- Convenience or prepared foods

- Microwave oven
- Dishwasher
- TV in the kitchen
- Takeout rotisserie chicken
- Pre-cut packaged vegetables
- Pre-washed bagged salads

So on this, one of Rose's typical days, she exercised (only she called it housekeeping, food shopping, doing the laundry, and ironing) for about six hours! That exercise included walking for at least thirty minutes and climbing at least two sets of stairs five times each. She ate three meals a day, which added up to about 1,600 calories, 38 percent fat (65 grams), and 20 grams of fiber. She got nine hours of sleep each night, and took a one-hour afternoon nap. Rose was happy with her life, contented with what she had, and wasn't looking for more than she needed.

Post script: Rose was a real person who lived a healthy life until she died of natural causes at 93.

Mary's Story

Mary is a forty-something new millennium supermom. She works as a full-time school administrator, is the mother of three children ages ten to eighteen years old, and close to earning her master's degree in education. Her husband works shifts and rotates different work schedules every month. Mary has had high blood pressure for several years; she also recently found out that she has high cholesterol and triglycerides. Mary has also struggled with her weight for several years. She's 5'1" and weighs 145 pounds. (Her BMI is 27, which classifies her as overweight.)

Morning

5:45–6:40: Gets up, puts in load of laundry, walks with a friend around neighborhood for about 40 minutes

6:40–8:10: Empties dishwasher, makes lunch for three kids, makes bed, gets ready for work, prepares breakfast for kids, eats breakfast herself, does whatever household chores time will allow (empty garbage, tidy up family room, or clip food coupons)

Breakfast: Two slices toast, 1 tbs. peanut butter, 4-oz. glass orange juice, peach

8:10–8:45: Drives youngest child to school, puts first load of laundry into dryer, starts second load, makes lunch to bring to work
8:45–9:00: Carpools with coworker
9:00–12:30: Observes class at one preschool

Afternoon

12:30–1:15: Lunch break

Lunch: Lettuce, 1/2 can water-packed tuna, 1 tbs. light dressing, orange, water

1:15–3:00: Writes observational report
3:00–3:20: Drops off coworker (if her turn to drive), returns home
3:20–4:00: Eats snack with daughter and helps her with her homework

Snack: Six low-fat cookies

4:00–5:00: Prepares dinner

Evening

5:00–6:00: Serves and eats dinner with whichever family members are home

Dinner: Two slices grilled chicken breast, large helping steamed broccoli with spray butter, large plain baked potato, water

6:00–8:30: Meets with graduate school study group three nights a week; grocery-shops two nights a week; works on graduate studies or school projects if at home

8:30–9:30: Eats a snack, calls elderly parent or friend (if she's not too tired)

Snack: Small cup of fat-free chocolate pudding

9:30–10:30: Puts the ten-year-old to bed, folds laundry, prepares clothes and books for next day

10:30: Goes to bed (husband may or may not be at home)

As you can see, Mary has put in a long, exhausting, stressful day by anyone's standards. She couldn't possibly have squeezed in any more activities—she had no time or energy left! After just seven hours of sleep, she forces herself to get up for that morning walk. Here's what she says about that exercise time: "I make myself do it because I have to get my weight, blood pressure, and cholesterol down and I know exercise will help. But do you know what? The whole time I'm walking I'm either thinking to myself of all I have to do as soon as I get back home or, even worse, I'm complaining to my friend!"

Mary takes in about 1,300 calories, 21 percent fat (30 grams) and 17 grams of fiber, and probably burned about 220 calories on her walk. She admits that before her most recent doctor visit, she wasn't watching her diet: "It's so much easier to order takeout or bring the kids to McDonald's. I don't have time or the energy to cook." She knows that she used food for comfort, so calories really didn't matter. High-fat, super-sized meals and snacks were the order of the day. But now she's proud of herself that she's walking and improving her diet.

Mary looks ahead to an easier daily pace. She admits, though, that taking it easy isn't in her immediate future: Her youngest child will be at home for several more years, her husband's erratic work schedule won't improve until he retires, and that's still many years away. She's concerned about her health;

she realizes that the stress in her life impacts that health. She'd like to slow down and smell the roses—if only she could find the magic to make it happen.

As crazy as Mary's life is, she's caught up in much the same vicious cycle that most of the rest of us are. Her daily doings show how today's lifestyle (and all the "conveniences" of it) can lead us down a slippery slope toward overweight and obesity. Here's how:

- Most of us eat too many calories, especially empty and high-fat calories. After all, it's easy to find cheap, unhealthful junk food just about anywhere, at any time, twenty-four hours a day, seven days a week. Worse yet, it's served in huge portions!
- Some of us go from eating too much to eating way too little, which also doesn't help us lose weight.
- Lots of us just aren't very active (where do you think the term "couch potato" comes from?).
- We're under way too much stress. It drains our energy and makes us feel tired, depressed, and sick.

The outlook seems pretty bleak, doesn't it? Isn't there *some* way you can take that overweight bull by its horns and put a stop to your weight gain and actually turn it around and start losing weight—for good? We're happy to say, the answer is yes! There's no magic involved, but if you're willing to think out of the *dieting* box, you could finally succeed at losing weight and keeping it off for the long haul.

The 10% Solution

Sure, *diet* is a four-letter word. But so are *love* and *good* and *life* and *food*. Goes to show you that four-letter words don't have to be "bad." When "diet" describes a way of eating, it can have a positive meaning, as in "a high-fiber *diet*" or "a balanced *diet.*" But "diet," as in diet -*ing*, isn't such a positive four-letter word. Why is that, if excess weight is such a health concern for so many of us? Shouldn't we "diet"? No—because those kinds of "diets" don't work. (Want proof? Ask any dieter!)

To lose weight and keep it off, you need to change your everyday habits. When you make gradual and reasonable changes, they become part of your lifestyle and don't feel like changes anymore. You won't feel deprived as new habits take hold because you won't feel as if you're sacrificing anything. It's just becomes the way you eat.

Losing just 10 percent of your current body weight—*no matter how overweight you are*—will reduce your risk factors for diabetes, heart disease, and some forms of cancer. Let's call it the "10% Solution." Losing just the first two digits of your total weight will give you more energy and a new start on a longer, healthier life. We list some examples of a 10 percent weight loss below.

- **Person 1:** 5'1" tall and weighs **145** lbs. 10% = losing **14.5 (14½)** lbs.
- **Person 2:** 5'5" tall and weighs **200** lbs. 10% = losing **20** lbs.
- **Person 3:** 5'8" and weighs **280** lbs. 10% = losing **28** lbs.
- **Person 4:** 6' tall and weighs **310** lbs. 10% = losing **31** lbs.

These examples prove that you don't have to lose all your extra weight to feel better and improve your health.

Did You Know . . . that obesity contributes to 325,000 deaths in the U.S. each year?

A True Story

Chris, a middle-aged man, is 5'9" tall and weighs 224 pounds (his BMI is 33, making him mildly obese). He takes medications for high blood pressure and high cholesterol; he also has type 2 diabetes but isn't on any medication yet. At a recent checkup, his doctor discovered that Chris's blood pressure was elevated and a fingerstick blood test revealed a high sugar reading. He talked to his doctor about what he should do: They agreed that Chris should lose some weight. The doctor suggested that Chris set up an appointment with a dietitian; he agreed, without enthusiasm.

Chris didn't want to keep his nutrition counseling appointment; after all, he thought he already knew what the dietitian would say to him: "I know what she is going to tell me. I have to eat smaller portions, not eat out, not have any ice cream, and, and, and . . ." but Chris did keep his appointment. And this is what the dietitian said to him:

"You weigh 224 pounds today. Will you consider losing just 10 percent of your present weight —that's 22 pounds—over the next six months? That's actually less than a pound a week. Once you've lost the 22 pounds, I'll teach you how to maintain that loss for another six months, which means that one year from now you'll weigh 200 pounds. When was the last time you weighed so little? And if you take six months to lose 22 pounds, then take another six months to maintain that loss, chances are very good that you'll stay at 200 pounds forever. That is, unless you decide to lose another 10 percent!"

The dietitian didn't tell Chris to lose 60 pounds. Instead, she suggested that he lose just 22, or 10 percent of his current body weight. Chris returned home feeling for the first time in his life that he really *could* lose those 22 pounds. He'd never felt so good about losing weight before. Ah-ha! *That* was the difference! After the dietitian outlined a meal plan for him and Chris realized that he had to work on just a few changes ("Work at your own pace," she said), he didn't feel overwhelmed and definitely didn't feel like he was "dieting."

After living with the 10% Solution/"I'm not dieting" attitude for nine weeks, Chris had lost seven pounds and was well on his way to achieving his own 10% Solution. Besides losing weight, Chris was also reducing his risk of developing heart disease as well as further diabetes complications. Chris knows that he still has a weight problem, and that he'll still be overweight even after he loses those 22 pounds. But he also knows he's improving his health with every pound he loses. In fact, he now says to himself, "I can do this!" His small but consistent *changes* are becoming *habits* and those *habits* are developing into a *lifestyle*—one that just happens to encourage weight loss and good health.

How the 10% Solution Can Be Sabotaged

So, your goal is to lose weight to improve your health, not to look good for a wedding or a reunion or so you can look better in your bathing suit on vacation. You decide to try to lose just 10 percent of your current weight over a relatively long period of time—twelve months, to be exact. What's the easiest way to make this approach work?

There's no way around it: To lose weight, the number of calories *coming in* has to be less than the number of calories *going out*. You can do this in three different ways:

1. You can cut back on the calories you eat (fewer calories *in*).
2. You can increase your amount of exercise (more calories *out*).
3. You can reduce the number of calories you're eating and exercise more (fewer calories *in* plus more calories *out*).

The problem is, if you go overboard and cut your calories too much and/or increase your exercise too much, before long you'll start feeling hungry and weak. You might even get dizzy or shaky or develop headaches. To make matters worse, you might also notice that you aren't even losing weight. What a drag! What's happening anyway?

Our bodies learned ages and ages ago, when our ancestors faced famines, to store as much energy as they possibly could. As we explained in Chapter 1, this is exactly what your body does with all excess calories; it turns them into body fat and that body fat becomes an energy reserve. Your body doesn't want to use its stored energy; in fact, it just wants to keep accumulating more and more (isn't *that* the truth?).

When the number of calories that you're taking *in* is much less than the calories you're putting *out*, alarms go off inside your body, forcing it to preserve its stored fat. Keep in mind that your body still has to come up with the energy it needs for all its necessary functions and activities. Since you aren't getting enough calories, you have to dig into your energy reserves to meet your energy needs. *Remember: Your body doesn't want to resort to this.* So, first it sends out some warnings: You may get a headache or feel faint. (These symptoms, by the way, signal low blood sugar, or hypoglycemia.) These indicators are your body's way of saying "Feed me. Give me the calories I need to keep enough energy pumping into those working cells."

If the warnings go unheeded, your body can still do something to prevent major energy losses from its fat stores. And here comes the bad news: It can simply slow down the rate at which it uses energy—the energy it needs to keep your heart pumping and continue performing all the other tasks it has to do to keep you alive. (The rate that your body uses energy for all its functions is called the *basal metabolic rate*.) Your body's doing only what it's learned to do throughout evolution: conserve energy.

Now, back to you, the dieter: What's happened? With all good intentions, you go on your "diet," which means that you're drastically cutting calories and exercising as much as you can. Yes, you feel horrible after a few days, but because you're determined to lose weight *this time,* you keep at it. You watch the scale and, after going down a pound or two or three, the needle stops moving. Wanting more spectacular results, you get frustrated and give up the "diet." You decide that you lack willpower, it's just too hard to lose weight, or there's something metabolically wrong with you, or all of the above. No—not true! There's nothing wrong with you, but a lot wrong with your approach to losing weight. What do you need to be convinced that *diets don't work?*

QUOTE OF THE DAY:
"I have not failed.
I've just found 10,000 ways that won't work."
—Thomas Edison

Tricklers and the 10% Solution

To succeed at losing weight, your body must work with you, not against you, during your deliberate energy shortage, more commonly known as a weight-loss diet. Your brain interprets how much energy it has to work with by the level of glucose in your blood. If enough calories aren't coming *in,* then the new supply of energy won't be enough. And as the glucose in your blood gets used up, your sugar level drops, and your brain interprets this drop as hunger. In other words, your brain wants you to eat more food so that it can receive a new supply of energy.

Your brain also registers hunger when there's a sharp rise in blood glucose followed by a rapid drop (which happens after lots of insulin activity), and reacts the same way it does when there's a calorie shortage, even when there isn't one. A large amount of insulin responds to the large amount of glucose in your blood. Unfortunately, you don't necessarily burn the glucose pulled out of your blood; if there's too much, you store it as fat. But because your blood-sugar level has been lowered, your brain wants you to eat more food so that it can renew its energy supply.

Question: What causes this continual hunger cycle?
Answer: Remember that your body breaks down gushers very quickly into glucose.

Question: Where does the glucose go?
Answer: From the small intestines into your bloodstream.

Question: What happens next?
Answer: Your brain tells your pancreas to secrete as much insulin as it needs at that time in order to accommodate the surge in blood sugar that resulted from the quickly digested gushers.

Question: Then what happens?
Answer: Your blood-sugar level drops quickly as insulin moves glucose from your blood to your cells.

Question: Is this blood-sugar roller-coaster good or bad?
Answer: It's bad if you're trying to lose weight, because now your body, thanks to your brain's alertness, goes into "preservation mode" to store as much energy as it can rather than burn as much energy as it can.

Question: Why does your body want to store energy?
Answer: Because it's afraid you'll starve: It's been preprogrammed to store as much glucose as it can when blood levels are low, regardless of *why* they're low.

Question: Can you prevent this from happening?
Answer: Yes!

Enter the tricklers, those slowly digested carbs that your body turns into glucose in a slow, steady way. By supplying a steady stream of glucose to the blood, which then sends this steady glucose supply to the working cells that are looking for it, your brain isn't registering hunger because your blood-sugar levels never dip low unless four or five hours have passed since you ate and it's time to eat again.

To succeed at losing weight, you can't feel hungry. Tricklers keep you from feeling hungry.

In order to lose weight and keep it off, you can't feel those energy highs and the inevitable lows (see above); instead, you need a consistent, steady supply of glucose to meet your endless energy needs. Tricklers, as you now know, are the best carb choices for keeping up a steady energy supply—even over a period of several hours. And when you keep getting the energy you need, those highs and lows are a thing of the past: You don't feel headachy or lightheaded, and you have plenty of energy to make it through the day and night. When your body gets what it needs from the food you eat, it's in harmony and gives you a great feeling of well being. Tricklers give you a sense of control. You can say to yourself, "Hey! I can do this!"

To succeed at losing weight, you need to feel good. Tricklers allow you to feel in control and enjoy a sense of well being.

You gradually have to use some of your fat stores in order to lose weight. By causing a slower, smaller, and steadier rise in blood-sugar levels, tricklers keep your body from pumping a surge of insulin into your bloodstream (see above). The result? Your cells will get just the right amount of sugar *as they need it*—no less and no more. Because if too much sugar dumps into your blood (and, as a result, too much insulin as well), what happens to the sugar that you don't need right then? Insulin delivers it to the liver, where it's converted into fat. This explains how gushers can add to fat stores, and why tricklers don't.

To succeed at losing weight, you must gradually use some of your stored fat. Tricklers help your body use this stored fat.

No food is bad. But the case remains strong: Carbohydrates are your body's fuel of choice. As you already know, in a healthy, balanced diet, the majority of your calories should come from carbohydrates. That's why carbohydrates are the single most influential nutrient you can eat; they affect your day-to-day living as well as your general health. To keep your weight under control, then, you need to look at the types of carbs you're eating. And tricklers (what we've also been calling slowly digested carbs, or low-G.I. carbohydrates) are the best types of carbs to help you lose weight and keep it off. You can take a peek at some low-G.I. meals and snacks by turning to page 150.

Are You Motivated to Lose Weight?

Did you know that the weakest motivator for shedding pounds is just *wanting* to? It's almost as if a little voice says, "Who are you trying to kid? Sure you'll be 'good' for a week or two, but come on; you know it's not going to work. Why should it? You've never kept lost weight off before!" After listening to that internal voice, who wouldn't feel defeated from the very start? On the other hand, you're strongly motivated to lose weight if you want to . . .

keep your good health. "Diabetes runs in my family. If I keep my weight down, I'll improve my odds of not getting it myself."

improve your health. "My doctor told me that if I could lose some weight, my blood pressure would improve and I might not need to take any medication."

boost your energy level. "If only I weren't so tired, maybe I could make dinner tonight and even go for a bike ride with the kids after school. But I'm exhausted. These extra 50 pounds I carry around all day long wear me out. I know that if I could lose some weight, I'd have more energy and feel younger too."

The Successful-Loser Profile

In 1994 the National Weight Control Registry began to track people who had lost weight and successfully kept it off for at least one year. To date, the registry has listed about 3,000 people ages eighteen and older who have maintained a weight loss of an average of thirty pounds. Here's how these successful weight losers did it:

> Eighty-nine percent watched their fat intake, controlled portion sizes, and burned an average of 400 calories a day, usually by walking.

To learn more about the National Weight Control Registry, call 1-800-606-NWCR (6927).

THE BOTTOM LINE

➤ More than 60 percent of American adults are overweight or obese.

➤ More than 70 percent of adults are dieting.

➤ More than 25 percent of American children (ages six to seventeen) are overweight.

➤ Losing just 10 percent of your extra weight will help you feel better and improve your health.

➤ Tricklers are the best types of carbs in a balanced diet to help you lose weight and keep it off.

Fiber-High Bran Muffins

THESE small muffins certainly pack a powerful energy punch. Top with a little dab of peanut butter and you're ready for several hours on the fast track.

《 Makes 48 muffins   Serving: 1 muffin 》

2 cups	boiling water
5 tsp.	baking soda
1 quart	low-fat buttermilk
¾ cup	margarine, room temperature
2 cups	sugar
2	eggs
½ cup	egg substitute
2 cups	bran flakes
4 cups	All Bran with Extra Fiber
5 cups	whole wheat flour
1 cup	walnuts, coarsely chopped
1 cup	dried blueberries (or 2 cups fresh), optional

1. Preheat oven to 425°. Spray 4 muffin tins with vegetable spray.
2. Pour boiling water into a medium-sized bowl, add in the baking soda, then buttermilk. Let cool.
3. Place margarine, sugar, eggs, and egg substitute in medium bowl. Beat for 2 minutes at medium speed until smooth.
4. Place both cereals in a food processor fitted with a steel blade. Process until coarsely ground.
5. Pour cereals into a large mixing bowl. Add in the flour.
6. Alternately add the buttermilk and creamed margarine mixture to the dry ingredients.
7. Fold in walnuts and fruit, if adding.
8. Bake 20 minutes.

EACH SERVING CONTAINS:
141 calories, 24 grams carbohydrate, 3 grams protein, 5 grams fat, 10 milligrams cholesterol, 4 grams fiber

G.I. = LOW–MODERATE

6

CONTROL YOUR BLOOD SUGAR THE GOOD-CARB WAY

Do you have diabetes? Chances are very good that if you don't, you know someone who does. In fact, most health experts agree. We're in the middle of an epidemic: In the last decade alone, the incidence of type 2 diabetes, by far the most common form of the disease, has shot up 40 percent! And among the thirty-something crowd, there's been an estimated 70 percent increase!

The word "epidemic" sounds both severe and scary, but is it accurate? Well, let's take a look at the facts:

- Every day, more than 2,000 people are diagnosed with diabetes, which adds up to almost 800,000 new cases every year.
- Sixteen million Americans have diabetes, but about one-third of them—almost 5½ million—don't know they have the disease because they have not yet been diagnosed.
- Diabetes took 64,751 American lives in 1998. (That's more people than died in the Vietnam War, which claimed 58,148 lives over a nine-year period.)
- Diabetes is the seventh leading cause of death in the U.S.

What Is Diabetes?

According to experts, diabetes is a chronic disease that makes a person incapable of breaking down and properly using the nutrients that result from food digestion either due to a lack of, or ineffective use of, insulin. You may remember that insulin escorts glucose, protein-building molecules, and fat-storing molecules (from carbohydrate, protein, and fat digestion, respectively) into cells to meet your ongoing energy and health maintenance needs.

Here's an easier way to describe the disease: If you have diabetes, your body isn't able to remove sugar (in the form of glucose, coming primarily from carbohydrate digestion) from your bloodstream and get it into your cells so they can use it for energy. This happens if you don't produce enough insulin or if your body uses it ineffectively. Without the right supply of insulin, blood levels of glucose, as well as the protein-building molecules (amino acids) and fat-storing molecules (fatty acids), will all rise. The amino acids and the fatty acids accumulate more slowly than glucose and will do so only after glucose levels are very high. The medical term for elevated blood-sugar levels is *hyperglycemia.*

> hyper = high
> glyc = sugar
> emia = blood

And so as fuel (food) enters your body and your gut digests those foods, glucose, amino acids, and fatty acids dump into your bloodstream. If your insulin supply either can't meet the glucose demand or the insulin just isn't working well as an escort, your glucose levels begin to rise very quickly. If these levels go high enough and stay that way for an extended period of time, the classic symptoms of high blood sugar, or *hyperglycemia,* show up, including fatigue, increased hunger, thirst, frequent urination, and unexplained weight loss. (We'll talk more about diabetes symptoms later in this chapter.)

Types of Diabetes

Diabetes can be classified into three different types, all of which are different diseases. People with any form of diabetes may experience some of the same telltale symptoms, however, and share common risk factors for prolonged complications.

Type 1 Diabetes

Type 1 diabetes used to be called insulin-dependent diabetes, or juvenile-onset diabetes. This form of the disease usually occurs before age thirty but can happen at any age. The classic symptoms of increased hunger and thirst, frequent urination, fatigue, and weight loss appear suddenly. You don't produce any insulin, so you must take daily insulin injections to survive. Five to 10 percent of people with diabetes have type 1.

Type 2 Diabetes

You may have heard type 2 diabetes referred to as non-insulin-dependent diabetes, or adult-onset diabetes. This type of diabetes usually occurs after age thirty but can also affect children and adolescents (a trend that's becoming more widespread as overweight and obesity rates for children and adolescents continue to rise). Ninety to 95 percent of people who have diabetes have type 2. The disease is more common in certain ethnic groups such as African Americans, Latinos, Native Americans, and Pacific Islanders. Overweight and obese people are at higher risk of type 2 diabetes.

If you have this form of the disease, you may not always show signs of hyperglycemia, such as blurred vision, numbness, and tingling in the hands and feet, slow wound healing, recurring yeast infections, and itchy skin. Sometimes you can control type 2 diabetes by making changes to your diet, although in addition to making dietary changes, some people may also need to take a pill or an insulin injection to control the disease.

Gestational Diabetes

Gestational diabetes (carbohydrate intolerance due to insulin resistance only during pregnancy) usually occurs between the 24th and 28th weeks of pregnancy and occurs in 2 to 5 percent of all pregnancies in the U.S. Women with gestational diabetes are considered at high risk, and since there may be no physical symptoms, a blood test is performed on all pregnant women. Although the disease disappears once the baby is born, many of these women may develop type 2 diabetes later on.

Impaired Glucose Tolerance

Health professionals are seeing more and more cases of impaired glucose tolerance, which in the past has been called borderline diabetes. People with this pre-diabetic condition may show no symptoms, but a blood test will provide the diagnosis. If you have impaired glucose tolerance, here's what your blood test results will show:

- fasting glucose test (110–125 mg/dl)
- oral glucose tolerance test (140–199 mg/dl)

Impaired glucose tolerance is a hallmark characteristic of a condition known as the metabolic syndrome (see Chapter 7). If left untreated, impaired glucose tolerance may develop into type 2 diabetes.

A Myth Dispelled

Question: If I eat too many sweets, will I get diabetes?
Answer: No.

Warning Signs of Diabetes

Type 1

➤ Extreme fatigue
➤ Unusual thirst
➤ Frequent urination
➤ Extreme hunger
➤ Unusual weight loss
➤ Irritability

Type 2

➤ Any type 1 symptoms
➤ Frequent infections
➤ Blurred vision
➤ Slow to heal cuts, bruises
➤ Tingling or numbness in hands or feet

Brain Teaser

Question: Which of the symptoms listed above do most people experience even before they're diagnosed with type 2 diabetes?
Answer: Tingling or numbness in hands or feet.

A Silent Killer

How can people have diabetes and not know it? Well, some people with type 2 diabetes may have no symptoms for a long time—maybe even years—or if they do, those symptoms are common enough to be explained away without much thought. Here are some of the disease's most common trademarks and how easy it would be to ignore them:

Extreme fatigue. *How you might ignore the sign:* "Sure I'm tired. But I put in a long day. And I'm not getting any younger." Because glucose isn't getting into your cells, they work on empty. Yet your cells need to keep working anyway, so you end up feeling tired.

Unusual thirst. *How you might ignore the sign:* "I've always been a big drinker. And anyway, I thought water was good for you." Getting more water is your body's attempt to dilute the concentrated amount of sugar in your blood. After all, your body would rather your blood be watery than syrupy.

Frequent urination, especially at night. *How you might ignore the sign:* "Doesn't everybody have to get up at least a few times during the night?" If you drink a lot of liquids because you're thirsty, you'll need to get rid of that liquid too.

Extreme appetite. *How you might ignore the sign:* "I must really be burning a lot of calories; I always seem to be hungry, even right after I've finished a meal." Because glucose isn't getting into your cells, your body thinks it needs more calories to get the glucose it needs and knows that it can get more calories by signaling you to eat more.

Unexplained weight loss. *How you might ignore the sign:* "So what? I have to lose weight anyway." As blood-sugar levels keep rising higher and higher, your body desperately tries to get rid of some glucose, so it does the unthinkable: It excretes it! The calories you lose in your urine make you lose weight.

The Scope of the Problem

It may be easy to dismiss diabetes symptoms, but ignoring them doesn't make them go away. In fact, once you have diabetes, it *never* goes away.

In addition to the staggering number of full-blown diabetes cases, some experts believe that as many as 20 or 30 million additional Americans may have an early form of type 2 diabetes "brewing" in their bodies. This early diabetes is also known as impaired glucose tolerance.

And as huge a problem as diabetes is among adults in this country, statistics show that the problem affects young people too: In fact, more and more children and adolescents are now being diagnosed with type 2 diabetes, which traditionally has been considered a disease of middle age. In the past five years alone, because of troubling overweight statistics, researchers have seen a tenfold increase in diabetes incidence in children. Childhood diabetes is a particular concern because the earlier the disease takes hold, the longer you'll need to ward off its complications.

The Diabetes Epidemic: Why Now?

You know the answer already: As a country, we eat too much and move around too little. In fact, it's no small wonder that Shape Up America!, a nonprofit organization that promotes healthy weight, coined the term "diabesity." The term stresses how important a trigger obesity is for the development of type 2 diabetes. And many of us also suffer from too much stress and fatigue.

But if these problems are so common, then why don't we all suffer from diabetes? Because only some people inherit a gene that makes the disease more likely to develop. For these people, the negative aspects of a fast-paced, computer-chipped, chocolate-chipped, potato-chipped, super-sized lifestyle may eventually get the better of them, and they succumb to diabetes.

How Does Diabetes Start?

No one really knows what causes diabetes, which is why there's still no cure for the disease. Advances in medical science keep improving our understanding of diabetes, though, and we certainly know a lot more now than we did eighty years ago, when insulin was a new discovery.

Question: What causes you to lose your ability to use glucose properly?

Answer: There are several possible causes of diabetes. Here are a few of them:

1. You could have inherited a gene that makes the disease more likely to develop
2. You may have been exposed to an environmental trigger such as stress, toxins, or a virus, which could cause your body to destroy its own insulin-making cells in the pancreas (called an autoimmune reaction)
3. Your cells could become resistant to insulin
4. Your pancreas could be secreting less insulin
5. Your liver could be producing too much glucose
6. Your diabetes could be caused by a combination of several of the factors listed above.

Who's at Risk for Diabetes?

You are at greater risk for developing type 1 diabetes if you have:

- ➤ A brother or sister with type 1
- ➤ At least one parent with type 1

You are at greater risk for developing type 2 diabetes if you:

- ➤ Have a family history of diabetes
- ➤ Are older than age forty-five
- ➤ Are overweight or obese, and are apple-shaped
- ➤ Are inactive
- ➤ Have high triglycerides
- ➤ Have low HDL (good) cholesterol
- ➤ Have had gestational diabetes or gave birth to a baby weighing nine or more pounds
- ➤ Are a member of certain racial and ethnic groups, such as an African American, Latino, Native American, Asian, and Pacific Islander

Carbohydrates: Good Guys or Bad Guys?

Since you need to eat to survive, it only makes sense that you would look to your diet for help in controlling diabetes. As you've read, if you're eating a healthy balanced diet, the majority of your calories should be coming from carbohydrates. Your body loves to break down carbs into glucose; it's easy, and your body gets lots of energy from little work. Remember, *carbohydrates are your body's fuel of choice*. That means that your body is willing to take every crumb or drop of any carbohydrate that you consume and break it down into glucose.

Hang on a minute, you say: If carbs most affect blood-sugar levels because they, more than any other kind of food, break down into glucose, doesn't that make them the nutritional bad guys for people with diabetes?

No. *No food is bad*. But the *type* of carbs you eat is all-important. Thanks to Glycemic Index research, we now know that even though all carbs wind up in your blood as sugar, some types of carbs get there sooner than others. And if you have diabetes, a steep, rapid rise (or gush) in blood glucose can present a real problem: If your body has trouble moving the sugar into your cells and too much remains in your blood, it can lead to serious problems for your eyes, your kidneys, your peripheral nerves, and your heart. That's bad.

So the bottom line is that while no food is bad, the quickly digested carbs that we've been calling gushers will make blood glucose control more difficult. They're not the bad guys, they're just, well, gushers!

Did You Know . . . that blood-sugar levels fluctuate all the time? It's perfectly normal for blood-sugar levels to rise 40 points after a meal.

Tricklers, the Superheroes

The more slowly glucose trickles into your blood, the easier it is for your body to manage the normal after-digestion sugar jump. If you've eaten slowly digested carbs, your body isn't overwhelmed with an onslaught of glucose molecules that should be moving from your blood into your cells, and the available insulin can better handle the small, steady flow of glucose from these slowly digested carbs.

So, here's the windup: With trickler carbs, glucose molecules enter your bloodstream gradually, then insulin slowly escorts them from your blood into your cells. And the pitch: While no food is bad, the slowly digested carbs that we call tricklers will make blood glucose control easier. And not only do tricklers help to control blood-sugar levels, they also provide you with fiber, vitamins, minerals, and phytochemicals that benefit the rest of your body too. Now, who wouldn't call these foods superheroes?

Do Tricklers Work in Real Life?

Babs, sixty-seven, mother of three and grandmother of six, has been married for forty-four years. She works as a full-time bookkeeper for the same small, family-owned sheet metal company where she has been employed for the past twenty-two years.

Babs is 5′4″; her weight has been steadily creeping up over the past several years to reach a record high of 229 pounds. (With a BMI of 39, she is moderately obese.) Because she carries her excess weight right around her middle, she is the perfect insulin-resistant "apple." (Studies show that excessive abdominal fat weakens insulin's ability to deliver glucose into the cells.) Twenty years ago, she was diagnosed with type 2 diabetes and started taking insulin three years later, after trying in vain to control her blood sugars with diet and pills. A biker and walker, Babs found herself becoming progressively more tired and wanting to do less and less physical activity. She was injecting herself with 25 units of insulin twice a day and saw blood-sugar readings ranging from 67 to 219, indicating poor blood-sugar control. She was also taking three medications to help control her high blood pressure.

Because Babs didn't know what she was doing wrong and didn't know how to make health improvements, she talked to her doctor and decided to get some nutritional counseling.

Babs's Diet: Before Carb Counseling

Breakfast: One-half grapefruit; 2 cups of regular coffee with half-and-half
Snack: Buttered roll; cup of regular coffee
Lunch: Small can tuna; 6 Triscuits; 12 oz. V-8 juice; 8 mini chocolate chip cookies
Snack: Orange
Dinner: Fried chicken breast; cup of rice with gravy; cup of tea
Snack: Three coconut macaroons

At first glance, Babs's diet doesn't seem too bad, does it? After all, she *did* eat two fruit servings, didn't she? And the tuna and the chicken breast are lean protein choices, right? And even though the V-8 is sky high in sodium, it's made of vegetables and they're good for you, right? Well, when you add them up, Babs ate about 2,300 calories a day, and 45 percent of them were coming from fats! Not good. Her average daily diet pretty much kept her at her current weight, but since Babs is already moderately obese, she needs to lose weight to become healthier. And because she continued to feel too tired to exercise, the stage was set for Babs to keep gaining weight, which would worsen her insulin resistance. Increased insulin resistance would, in turn, continue to raise her blood-sugar levels, leaving her feeling hungry and tired, and continuing the vicious cycle.

How Could Babs Improve Her Diet?

The first thing Babs could do to help herself would be to start her day with a well-balanced breakfast, which would rev up her "motor" and start her burning as many calories as possible from the very beginning of the day. Then, by reducing her fat intake and introducing more tricklers into her diet (especially by eating whole grain breads and crackers, and including vegetables and low-fat dairy products), Babs's blood-sugar levels would stabilize and she wouldn't feel so hungry. She would feel satisfied with fewer calories and would eat less. The result? Babs should start to lose weight and gradually become less insulin resistant. Both of these changes would improve her blood-sugar control as well as her quality of life.

Babs's Diet: After Carb Counseling

Breakfast: One cup old-fashioned oats cooked in cup of 1% milk; ½ cup natural applesauce; regular coffee with fat-free half-and-half

Snack: Four Social Tea biscuits; decaf coffee

Lunch: Two oz. lean roast beef sandwich on 2 slices 100% stoneground whole-wheat bread with lettuce, tomato, and mustard; a sandwich-sized Baggie of cut-up raw vegetables; water

Snack: Eight oz. light yogurt; ¾ cup honeydew and cantaloupe

Dinner: Three oz. grilled salmon; cup mashed sweet potatoes; 2 cups broccoli; small baked apple with cinnamon

Snack: Four oz. 1% milk; oatmeal cookie

It's hard to believe: All the food in Babs's "after" diet adds up to 600 *fewer* calories than her previous day's diet. The amounts of fruits and vegetables, dairy servings, and high-fiber, slowly digested tricklers increased as her fat and calorie intake greatly decreased. The after diet amounts to 1,700 calories, and 24 percent fat.

Babs: Down 20 and Feeling Great!

After just four months of dietary changes, Babs lost twenty pounds. (With another three-pound weight loss, she will have reduced her body weight by 10 percent—the 10% Solution.) After losing those last three pounds, she'll learn how to maintain that loss for several more months, then may decide to lose more weight. And that terrific weight-loss success has brought with it some wonderful health benefits (didn't we tell you it would?): Babs no longer needs *any* insulin injections and her doctor has reduced her oral diabetes medication too. Her blood sugars have stabilized and now fall completely within the normal range. Another bonus: Because of her weight loss, Babs's blood pressure has returned to normal and her doctor may reduce her levels of those medications too.

So all of the health conditions that have caused Babs so much trouble over the years have quickly improved: Her weight, blood sugars, and blood pressure have all plummeted. The only thing that hasn't taken a nosedive is her spirits: "When I was too tired to do anything, I just didn't know who I was anymore. Now I feel really great—just like a teenager!"

Babs offers further proof that eating a healthful, balanced diet that's full of low-G.I. foods works in real life!

THE BOTTOM LINE

➤ If you don't produce enough insulin or use it ineffectively, you will likely develop diabetes.

➤ There are three types of diabetes: type 1, type 2, and gestational.

➤ Doctors are seeing more people with "impaired glucose tolerance," a pre-diabetic condition that results from excess weight and obesity.

➤ Quickly digested carbs, gushers, make blood-glucose control more difficult.

➤ Slowly digested carbs, tricklers, make blood-glucose control easier.

Saffron Rice Pilaf

THIS colorful rice dish blends flavorful ingredients into a definite crowd-pleaser.

❮ **Makes 4 cups   Serving size: ½ cup** ❯

½ tbs.	olive oil
Small	onion, finely chopped
2 cloves	garlic, minced
1 cup	Uncle Ben's Converted Rice
Dash	saffron threads
2½ cups	hot broth (chicken or vegetable)
1 tsp.	salt (omit if broth is not low sodium)
2 tbs.	fresh parsley (4 sprigs), finely chopped

1. Heat oil in a medium saucepan over medium heat. Add the onion and sauté until soft, about 4 to 5 minutes.
2. Add the garlic and sauté for another 2 minutes (do not let garlic turn brown).
3. Add the rice and saffron and stir to coat with the oil.
4. Add the hot broth and salt (if used) and stir gently. Reduce heat and cover.
5. Simmer for 20 minutes.
6. Remove from heat; let rest for 5 minutes.
7. Add parsley. Fluff rice with fork and serve.

EACH SERVING CONTAINS:
97 calories, 20 grams carbohydrate, 2 grams protein, 1 gram fat, 0 milligrams cholesterol, 2 grams fiber

G.I. = LOW

7

GOOD CARBS: YOUR KEY TO A HEALTHIER HEART

Did you know that coronary heart disease, or CHD, is the number-one killer of men and women in the U.S.? In fact, more than a half million Americans die each year from heart attacks caused by CHD. And high blood pressure, a risk factor for heart disease, affects 50 million Americans—that's about 20 percent of the entire population. (About one-third of these people don't even know that their blood pressure is high.) Here are some more sobering statistics:

- The prevalence of high blood pressure in African Americans is among the highest in the world.
- Heart disease is the leading cause of death in American women.
- About 60 percent of all Americans age sixty and older have high blood pressure.
- About 7 million Americans suffer from coronary heart disease, the most common form of heart disease.
- Every twenty-nine seconds an American has a heart attack or goes into cardiac arrest.

Now here's some better news:

- Because of new screening guidelines, about 65 million Americans will be treated for high cholesterol and about 36 million will take cholesterol-lowering medication.

- Research has proven that lowering LDL ("bad") cholesterol levels can reduce the risk for short-term heart disease by as much as 40 percent.
- Between 1983 and 1995, the percentage of the public who had ever had their cholesterol checked rose from 35 percent to 75 percent.
- Since 1978, average total cholesterol levels dropped 10 points from 213 mg/dl to 203 mg/dl.

So the message is: Heart disease kills but it doesn't have to kill *you*. That is, as long as you go for regular checkups, eat a healthful diet, exercise, and take proper care of yourself. That's a start, right?

What Is Coronary Heart Disease?

Coronary heart disease results from the narrowing of one or both of the coronary arteries that feed oxygen, and energy as glucose to your heart. Over time, your arteries become hard and stiff. Although physicians call this narrowing *atherosclerosis*, most of us know it as hardening of the arteries. People used to think that atherosclerosis was just a natural consequence of growing older, but the chronic buildup of plaque and the resulting hardened arteries and decreased, even blocked, blood flow to the heart is showing up even among young people in the prime of their lives! We know this because the incidence of heart attacks, high blood pressure, angina, and other related conditions is rising, even among young people.

What Narrows Arteries?

Arteries become narrow when there's a buildup of plaque, deposits that are made mostly of cholesterol and some other fats and cells. If you have a lot of cholesterol in your blood, these deposits get bigger over time and narrow the arteries' passageway. That narrowing eventually reduces blood flow to your heart, which needs an uninterrupted supply of food and oxygen to function properly. Too much cholesterol blocks arteries and can cause heart pain (angina) or a heart attack.

What can cause an artery to become completely clogged? A lot of plaque buildup or a large blood clot. (Blood clots are more likely to form in arteries with heavy plaque buildup.) Any way you look at it, whether it's because of clogging or clotting, cholesterol is usually at least partly to blame.

Are You at Risk?

Several factors contribute to your heart disease risk, many of which you can control by eating well and getting more exercise. (We'll talk more about that later in this chapter.) Two risk factors, though, your genes and your age, you can do nothing about.

It runs in the family. If heart disease affects other members of your family, you, too, may have inherited the same genetic tendency as some of your relatives. If your father or brother had premature heart disease (before age fifty-five) or your mother or sister had heart disease (before age sixty-five), there's a strong possibility that you have inherited this risk factor.

You're getting older. Once men reach age forty-five and women reach fifty-five, their age becomes a risk factor for heart disease. And no matter how many fountain-of-youth products you use—from skin creams to cosmetic surgery—nothing can change your body's age.

The Risk Factors You Can Control

You can improve your heart health by focusing on those risk factors you *can* control: cholesterol, blood pressure, elevated blood sugars, weight, smoking, and stress (notice how many of these factors are diet-related). Here are nine strategies to work into your new, healthful lifestyle:

Heart-Health Strategy #1:
Lower Total and LDL (Bad) Cholesterol

According to experts, your total cholesterol number is high if it's above 200 mg/dl and your levels of LDL ("bad") cholesterol are high if they are greater than 130 mg/dl. (Cholesterol levels are measured in milligrams [mg] of cholesterol per deciliter [dl] of blood.) Here's how to reduce both total and LDL cholesterol numbers:

Limit amounts of high-fat animal products. Some fatty foods include spare ribs, sausage, hot dogs, burgers, bacon, salami, bologna, butter, whole-milk cheese, and whole-milk products.

Limit saturated fats. Sometimes we don't know that we're even eating saturated fats because they're hidden in prepared foods such as pastries, cookies, pies, gravies, and cream sauces. Eat these foods in moderation if at all.

Avoid trans fats. You can recognize trans fats if you read something such as "partially hydrogenated vegetable oil" on the food's ingredient list. Some foods that may contain trans fats include shortening, margarines, crackers, and cookies.

Cook the low-fat way. Bake, broil, grill, or steam your foods. For new ideas, buy a health magazine that includes recipes or surf the Web for some low-fat recipes to try.

Eat more high-fiber foods. Some high-fiber superstars include vegetables, fruits, and whole grains—tricklers!

> *Did You Know. . .* Foods derived from plants such as grains, cereals, fruits, and vegetables don't contain cholesterol. Only animals and foods made from animals contain cholesterol.

Heart-Health Strategy #2:
Increase HDL (Good) Cholesterol

Because HDL cholesterol protects against heart disease, the higher the number, the better. A level less than 40 mg/dl is low and is considered a major risk factor because it increases your risk for developing heart disease. If your levels are a bit on the low side, here's how you can pull them up:

Include monounsaturated and omega 3 fats in your daily diet. They help to protect your HDL levels. Keep in mind, though, that overdoing it won't give you extra protection, just extra calories. Good sources of monos include olive and canola oils, avocado, natural unsalted peanut butter, peanuts, and almonds. And good sources of omega 3 fats include salmon, white albacore tuna, sardines, flaxseed, and walnuts.

Get more exercise. Research shows that exercise can boost levels of this good cholesterol.

Stop smoking. Cigarette smoking, already a risk factor for heart disease, can also bring good cholesterol levels down. (It's never too late to kick the habit.)

The National Cholesterol Education Program Cholesterol Guidelines for Non-Diabetics

Total Cholesterol Number	Category
Less than 200 mg/dl*	Desirable
200–239 mg/dl	Borderline high
240 mg/dl and above	High

*Cholesterol levels are measured in milligrams (mg) of cholesterol per deciliter (dl) of blood.

LDL Cholesterol Number	Category
Less than 100 mg/dl	Optimal
100–129 mg/dl	Near optimal/above optimal

130–159 mg/dl	Borderline high
160–189 mg/dl	High
190 mg/dl and above	Very high

HDL Number Affect on Heart Disease Risk

Less than 40 mg/dl	Increases risk
60 mg/dl or higher	Helps lower risk

True or false: Cholesterol supplies you with lots of calories. **False.** Cholesterol provides no calories at all. Why? Because you can't break down cholesterol as you do carbohydrates, protein, and fat, so you don't get any energy from it.

The National Cholesterol Education Program Cholesterol Guidelines for Diabetics

	Low	Borderline	High
LDL	less than 100	100–129	130 or higher
HDL	greater than 45	35–45	less than 35
Triglycerides	less than 200	200–399	400 or higher

Heart Disease Risk: Triglycerides

Triglycerides are stored blood fats, and their levels fluctuate throughout the day. High-fat or excessively high-carbohydrate meals, excessive amounts of alcohol, sickness, and stress can all raise triglyceride levels.

What's a normal triglyceride reading? According to the National Heart, Lung, and Blood Institute, your triglyceride number should be below 200. Many doctors, though, try to get their patients' levels below 150 or even 100.

Heart-Health Strategy #3:
Lower High Blood Pressure

Your blood pressure is normal if your numbers are no higher than 140/90 (or no higher than 130/80 if you have diabetes). To lower your blood pressure, try these techniques:

Achieve and maintain a healthy weight. Overweight people are at greater risk for developing high blood pressure.

Become more physically active. Exercise not only can help you avoid high blood pressure altogether, it can also help you lower it if you already have the condition. Be sure to check with your doctor first if you haven't exercised for awhile or want to start an exercise program.

Eat a balanced diet loaded with tricklers. Because they are high in nutrients, including fiber, low-G.I. foods such as fruits, vegetables, and whole grains can help keep your blood pressure low.

Choose and prepare foods with less salt. If you have high blood pressure or are salt sensitive, you can reduce your risk by following the American Heart Association's recommendation to limit your salt intake to no more than 1$\frac{1}{4}$ teaspoons a day.

Drink alcoholic beverages in moderation. Drinking too much alcohol can cause blood pressure levels to rise, whether you actually suffer from high blood pressure or not. So be good to yourself and drink only in moderation. (That's good advice for everyone.)

Heart-Health Strategy #4:
Control Diabetes

Scientists have identified diabetes as an independent risk factor for heart disease; that is, even if you don't have any other risk factors, you're still in danger of developing heart disease simply because you have diabetes. (We explain an associated problem, the Metabolic Syndrome, which involves insulin resistance and carries a serious risk for heart disease, at length below. See "Do You Have the Metabolic Syndrome?" on this page.) To find out if you have diabetes, and to treat it properly if you do, follow these guidelines:

Get tested. See your doctor, get the prescribed lab work done, and discuss the results with him/her.

Prioritize your medical concerns. Are your blood sugars too high? Maybe your LDL cholesterol is off the charts? Are you overweight? Whatever concerns you may have, decide with your doctor which you should tackle first.

Work with your doctor and a registered dietitian. These health professionals will help you develop a game plan to address your needs. Chances are, you'll receive a meal plan that will improve your diet-related risk factors. And guess which type of diet works best? You guessed it: A balanced, high-carb, low-G.I. diet, with appropriate amounts of heart-healthful proteins and fats. A steady diet of these kinds of healthful foods have been proven to lower cholesterol, lower blood sugar, and promote gradual weight loss, which also improves blood pressure.

Start exercising. There's no need to do anything special; walking is fine. After all, you need no special equipment, and you can do it anytime, anywhere. If you haven't exercised for awhile or want to start an exercise program, always check with your doctor first. That's especially important advice if you have diabetes, because your doctor may have special instructions.

Do You Have the Metabolic Syndrome?

The Metabolic Syndrome describes a cluster of heart disease risk factors. Here's how to tell if you might have it: Do you have high blood pressure? Low HDL levels? High triglycerides? Has your doctor told you that you're insulin resistant? Are you apple-shaped, carrying your excess weight around your middle? If you answered yes to four or five of these questions, you're likely to have the metabolic syndrome. Just two or three yes answers? In time, you could develop the syndrome.

Apple shape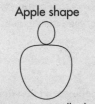

Pear shape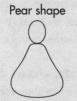

larger waist, smaller hips   smaller waist, larger hips

There is significant health benefit in reducing your waist measurement, particularly if you have an "apple" shape.

For several years, this cluster of risk factors was called Syndrome X because doctors didn't clearly understand what was happening in people with these characteristics. It was a hot topic among endocrinologists, doctors who specialize in metabolic diseases. Since then, research has shown that Syndrome X is, in fact, a genetic metabolic disorder that puts a person at high risk for heart disease. So now it has become a hot topic for cardiologists too. In fact, medical professionals now carefully monitor a growing number of patients who exhibit this cluster of symptoms.

Here's what is going on: If you're insulin resistant, your pancreas secretes enough insulin to meet your body's glucose load, but your cells are uncooperative or resistant to the insulin. So as glucose keeps pouring into your blood from the food that you're digesting, your pancreas just keeps secreting more and more insulin. All this extra insulin manages to keep blood glucose levels within the normal range, but usually at the high end of normal.

Insulin resistance by itself does not cause diabetes, although some people with diabetes are also insulin resistant (witness Babs in Chapter 6). But insulin resistance does lead to chronically high insulin levels. And those high insulin levels lead to high triglycerides, low HDL (good) cholesterol, and high blood pressure—all known risk factors for heart disease.

The good news: Studies have shown that certain types of carbohydrates (yes, the tricklers) increase insulin sensitivity, which decreases insulin resistance.

And This Just In . . .

New research shows that chronic sleep deprivation may contribute to insulin resistance. So how much sleep do you need? More than six and a half hours each night.

Heart-Health Strategy #5: Lose Weight

You already know that diets don't work. Here's a rundown of some of the changes you need to make to take off that extra weight, reduce your risk of heart disease, and look and feel great at the same time.

Modify your diet. Gradually these positive changes will become habits that will last a lifetime. And these habits will be based on improving your health, not losing weight. Losing weight will be a fringe benefit!

Eat three balanced meals a day. Eating meals—as well as one to three snacks during the day—will keep you from getting too hungry by keeping your blood-sugar levels relatively constant.

Don't drastically cut calories. Most women can lose weight eating 1,400 calories a day; most men eating 1,700 to 1,800 calories a day.

Heart-Health Strategy #6:
Eat More Trickler Carbs as Part of a Balanced Diet

One of the easiest and most heart-healthful lifestyle changes that you can make is to incorporate more slowly digested carbs (low-G.I. carbs, or tricklers) into your daily diet. (This change ties in with the other heart-health strategies too, so you can address several of them at once.) Trickler carbs include whole-grain cereals, breads, and crackers, minimally processed flours and other starches, as well as most fruits and vegetables.

The remaining foods that you eat should be healthful protein- and fat-containing foods. You can refer back to the Food Guide Pyramid for recommendations by turning to page 7.

In addition, a heart-healthful balanced diet will be low in saturated fat and cholesterol. Limiting these dietary fats will make a huge dent in lowering your LDL (bad) cholesterol and help prevent hardening of the arteries from plaque buildup. That means limiting your portions of high-fat foods, including but not limited to, fatty or greasy meats, butter, cream sauces and gravies, bakery products, deep-fried foods, non-fat-reduced cheese, and whole-milk products. Keep in mind that you don't have to stop eating these foods completely—no food is bad—just eat smaller portions, and have them less often.

A heart-healthful balanced diet will also be high in fiber. Fiber in your gut helps to lower LDL cholesterol and tri-glycerides. Which foods are high in fiber? Carbohydrates such as whole grain breads and cereals, fruits, and vegetables. You may have already guessed the kinds of heart-healthful carbs we're talking about: tricklers!

Scientific Proof for Carbs

Several recent studies have shown that trickler carbs can help reduce heart disease risk. Other studies have shown that these same slowly digested carbs also reduce levels of total cholesterol, triglycerides, and boost levels of healthy HDL cholesterol.

A June 2000 study confirmed the heart-health benefits of slowly digested tricklers. The results came from the famous Nurses' Health Study, which has been tracking the medical histories and lifestyles of more than 120,000 women since 1976.

This particular study looked at how the type of carbohydrates that 75,000 people consumed affected their risk for coronary heart disease. The researchers were comparing high and low Glycemic Index carbs, in other words, gushers and tricklers.

After looking at thousands of food questionnaires, the investigators found that surges of glucose into the blood (from the digestion of refined carbohydrates) increased the risk of coronary heart disease, especially in overweight people.

These findings have brought into question the soundness of what scientists have been recommending for years: that to reduce heart disease risk, you should eat a low-fat, high-carbohydrate diet. These new findings, along with the knowledge that too much circulating insulin can have a negative impact on heart health, should encourage health authorities to spell out the *type* of carbohydrates we should be eating. Here's what a more precise dietary recommendation for heart health might look like:

"Eat a balanced diet that consists of *high-fiber, slowly digested (low-G.I., or trickler) carbohydrates* with a low to moderate amount of fat, in which saturated fat and cholesterol are minimal and monounsaturated and polyunsaturated fats are eaten in moderation."

Heart-Health Strategy #7: Stop Smoking

Smoking raises your blood pressure and heart rate, lowers levels of good cholesterol, and increases your risk of developing blood clots that can lead to a heart attack. Worse yet, according to the American Heart Association, smoking is the biggest risk factor for sudden cardiac death. To help you kick the habit, try these tips:

Talk to your doctor. From patches to gums to medication, your doctor has lots of options to help you kick the habit.

Join a smoking cessation support group. That extra help and support may be just what you need to quit smoking for good.

Don't fear weight gain. Sure, you burn slightly fewer calories at rest once the nicotine leaves your system. But most of the weight comes from what you put in your mouth *in place of* the cigarette—candy, cookies, chocolates, crackers, plain bagels—all gushers, which make you eat more! So start eating trickler foods *now* to prevent weight gain when you decide to quit smoking.

Shed the Expense

Remind yourself that the four dollars you spend on cigarettes could buy a bouquet of flowers or a half-pound of decaf gourmet coffee instead.

Heart-Health Strategy #8:
Become More Physically Active

As busy as we all are, sometimes it's hard to find enough time to exercise or stay motivated to keep at it. To help you out, here are some exercise tips, many of them from the President's Council on Physical Fitness and Sports:

Check with your doctor first. If you're just starting an exercise program or haven't been active for awhile, get your doctor's okay first to be sure it's safe.

Make exercise a part of your daily routine. Set a regular time to exercise each day and stick to it. If you have workout time written on your calendar, you'll be more likely to keep the "appointment."

Start gradually. Start out slowly—about five to ten minutes at first; then increase your time to thirty to sixty minutes.

Invite a friend to join you. You'll be more likely to exercise regularly if you work out with a friend.

Rest when you need to. You aren't competing with anyone; you're exercising to stay healthy. So take a break when you need it. But if you've been exercising vigorously, don't stop suddenly or you may feel dizzy or faint.

Drink lots of water. Be sure to drink lots of water before, during, and after you exercise. Don't wait until you're thirsty.

Keep a daily written record of your progress. Tracking your progress, whether it's miles walked or time spent lifting weights, can work motivational miracles.

Exercise to your favorite music. Dance around the living room or take a walk with your personal tape player. (Keep the volume low enough, though, that you can hear all the sounds around you.)

Look for distraction. If you really don't like to exercise, ride a stationary bike, walk on a treadmill, or lift weights while watching your favorite TV show or movie. Before you know it, your time will be up!

Wear comfy clothing. The more comfortable you are, the more likely you are to enjoy physical activity.

Heart-Health Strategy #9: Manage Stress

Seems like we're rushing around all day, every day—from work meetings to after-work meetings, to kids' soccer practice and music lessons. Leading a stress-free life seems like an impossible dream. Luckily, there are some things you can do to *manage* the stress you have. Here are a few tips:

Accept that stress exists. You may find it comforting to realize that stress is just a part of life and that we're all in the same boat.

Name your stress. Giving your stress a name—whether it's your work schedule, family problems, medical worries, being overweight, or caring for an elderly parent—can help you better identify the problem and find solutions.

Identify your control. Try to determine which stresses you can do something about and look for ways to break down larger problems into several little ones that you can do something about. Then tackle your concerns one at a time.

Build a support network. You don't have to go it alone. Call on friends and family members to help you through tough times or just to listen. And keep in mind that some stresses may require professional help.

Eat trickler carbs. These slowly digested foods will keep you off the sugar roller-coaster and help you to feel energetic instead of drained. When you feel peppier, you'll also feel more in control and have a better sense of well-being.

Low Saturated Fat + Low Glycemic Index Carbs (Tricklers) = Heart Health

Here's the rundown of how to eat for optimum heart health:

- ▶ Eat a well-balanced diet.
- ▶ Eat 50 to 60 percent of total daily calories from carbohydrate foods.
- ▶ Make most carbohydrate choices the slowly-digested, low-G.I. trickler kind.
- ▶ Limit fat calories to 25 to 35 percent of total calories.
- ▶ Reduce your daily intake of saturated fat to less than 7 percent of total calories.
- ▶ Make most of the fats you eat polyunsaturated and monounsaturated.
- ▶ Consume less than 200 milligrams of cholesterol a day.
- ▶ Gradually increase your fiber intake to 20 to 30 grams a day.

True Stories from the Healthy Hearts Club

Marty's Story

Marty is a fifty-six-year-old full-time college professor. He is 5′9″ and weighs 237 pounds (BMI of 35, or moderately obese). Divorced for the past fifteen years, Marty lives alone and faithfully incorporates a twenty-minute walk into his daily routine; he also tries to play basketball once or twice a week. Marty skips breakfast during the week and picks up lunch between classes. He prepares many of his evening meals at home. When he was forty-three, Marty had a heart attack. Since placing him on cholesterol-lowering medication, his cardiologist has been pleased with the results of Marty's annual blood work. During his last physical, however, Marty's blood pressure was slightly elevated and his fasting blood sugar was above normal.

Marty's Diet: Before Carb Counseling

Breakfast: Four mugs regular black coffee (between 6 and 10 A.M.)

Lunch: Hamburger, medium fries, diet Coke

Snack: Diet Coke

Dinner: Twelve-oz. steak, half a restaurant portion of fettuccine alfredo, salad, water

Marty's diet made him a second heart attack waiting to happen. He eats too many calories (about 2,600 a day), and his diet is too high in fats and sodium and too low in fiber. Worse yet, Marty typically eats at least half of his calories late in the evening. His unhealthy dietary habits just couldn't be offset by his daily twenty-minute walk and the occasional basketball game and lacks three nutrient heavyweights: fruits, vegetables, and low-fat dairy foods. His elevated blood pressure and moderate obesity are directly affected by the way he eats.

Marty proves that cholesterol-lowering medication isn't the complete remedy for heart health; he needs to make some lifestyle changes too, such as improving his diet, getting more exercise, and managing his stress.

Marty says that he's never hungry, probably because of all the fat he eats—about 1,500 calories worth on an average day. He knows his diet is unhealthful, but he doesn't know how to change it.

How Could Marty Improve His Diet?

To start eating a more healthful and more balanced diet, Marty could eat a breakfast that consists of a low-G.I. whole grain bread or cereal, non-fat milk, and fruit. A turkey sandwich on rye with a salad and a piece of fruit would be easy to find in the cafeteria, he admitted. His new rule-of-thumb for dinner, whether at home or eating out, could be to fill half of his plate with vegetables; then his portions of starch and protein, the foods with more calories, would be controlled automatically.

Marty's Diet: After Carb Counseling

Breakfast: Half a pumpernickel bagel with natural, no-salt-added peanut butter and all-fruit jelly, 1 mug of coffee

Snack: A bowl of Special K with a cup skim milk, ¼ cantaloupe

Lunch: (brought from home) reduced-fat cheese and roasted pepper sandwich on rye, pear, water

Snack (two to three times a week): No-sugar-added hot chocolate, 2 to 3 graham crackers

Dinner: One cup steamed brown rice, 2 cups steamed vegetables, small grilled chicken breast, water

Snack: Handful of grapes

Seems like a lot of food, doesn't it? Would you believe that Marty's new diet contains about 750 fewer calories than before? He also cut his fat intake by 70 percent!

Marty's New Diet Serves Up Success

Marty actually liked eating this new way and found it easy to make the changes. And his results speak for themselves: After six months, he had lost twenty-three pounds! (Ten percent of his body weight—the 10% Solution.) In addition to playing basketball once or twice a week, he started playing golf and softball, and also found time to walk on his treadmill every day. As a result of these changes, his blood pressure is now normal, and his fasting blood-sugar level has dropped 35 percent, putting it back in the normal range.

Will Marty continue to eat heart-healthy meals and exercise? Here's his answer: "Eating low-fat, high-fiber meals isn't hard to do at all. Not only do I feel good, but also my doctor tells me to keep at it, because the changes are working. I can do that!"

Marco's Story

Marco provides another example of how changes can become habits that turn into a healthy lifestyle. Marco, a fifty-six-year-old man of Hispanic descent, works full-time for a news agency. He is 5'9" and weighs 232 pounds (BMI of 34, mildly obese). At fifty-four, he was diagnosed with type 2 diabetes, which he controlled by taking two pills a day. He also has mildly elevated blood pressure, which no medication seemed able to improve. His most recent blood work showed that he has elevated cholesterol. A nonsmoker who occasionally drinks a glass of wine with dinner, Marco tries to walk a mile around his complex three times a week, which takes him twenty minutes. He complains of feeling tired and hungry most days.

Marco's Diet: Before Carb Counseling

Breakfast: Four cups regular coffee with 2% milk, bagel with cream cheese

Lunch: Tuna salad on rye, Manhattan clam chowder, few saltines, diet Pepsi

Snacks (throughout the day): Chips, cookies, pretzels, diet iced tea

Dinner: Pot roast, pan-fried potatoes, steamed broccoli, escarole sautéed in olive oil, tomato and onion salad, blue cheese dressing, glass of wine

Marco's meals sound fairly typical: They're full of calories and loaded with fat. This high-fat eating style contributed to his mild obesity, and his excess weight negatively affected his diabetes, cholesterol, and blood pressure. And to make matters worse, Marco spent his day on caffeine overload. His twenty-minute walk every other day was a step in the right direction, but only a small one.

How Could Marco Improve His Diet?

A close look at Marco's diet shows that he was eating only about 30 percent of his daily calories from carbohydrates, and the carbs he chose had high-G.I. values: bagels, saltines, potatoes, pretzels. Along with the steady flow of caffeine (from drinks such as coffee, diet Pepsi, and diet iced tea), these gusher carbs elevated his blood sugar and stimulated his appetite. If he can start choosing whole-grain breads and crackers and some lower-G.I. cooked grains such as pasta or long-grain rice, and if he can reduce his caffeine intake, he'll start feeling more satisfied with fewer calories. Over time his blood sugar, cholesterol, blood pressure, and weight should all go down. He'll also have a lot more energy.

Marco's Diet: After Carb Counseling

Breakfast: Bowl of All-Bran with Extra Fiber, one cup skim milk, a Granny Smith apple, decaf coffee

Lunch: Large garden salad with grilled chicken breast, low-fat balsamic vinaigrette dressing, one pita bread, dish fresh strawberries, sparkling water

Snack: A handful of sourdough pretzel nuggets

Dinner: Two tilapia filets poached in white wine, ear of corn, steamed asparagus, tomato and onion salad with grated cheese, oil, and vinegar, small bunch red grapes, decaf diet soda

Marco's Small Changes Yield Big Results

After just five months of a few diet and exercise changes, Marco lost 25 pounds—enough that his doctor was able to discontinue all his diabetes and blood pressure medications, since his levels had returned to normal. After eighteen months, Marco continued to maintain his new weight of 209 pounds, which is down 23 pounds from his original weight, and slightly more than 10 percent of his total weight. His blood sugar, blood pressure, and cholesterol values stayed normal—all without prescribed medications. Truly, Marco has followed Hippocrates' advice: "Let thy food be thy medicine." This is what he thinks of himself now: "It's unbelievable how good I feel. Not only am I walking every day, but also I jog half the way! I've never had so much stamina!"

THE BOTTOM LINE

➤ Heart disease is the number one killer of American men and women. But if you control your risk factors, it doesn't have to kill you.

➤ You can reduce your risk of heart disease and high blood pressure by eating a balanced diet loaded with trickler carbs, heart-healthful proteins and fats.

➤ To reduce heart attack risk you should also:

➤ lower your blood pressure if it's high

➤ reduce levels of total and LDL cholesterol

➤ increase HDL cholesterol

➤ lose weight if you're overweight

➤ find out if you have diabetes and control it if you do

➤ quit smoking

➤ exercise for at least 30 minutes every day

➤ manage stress

➤ A healthful diet comes from healthful eating habits. You may still need medication to manage your heart disease risk factors, but why not help yourself by letting food also serve as your medicine?

Just-Plain-Good Pasta

IF you like natural, earthy flavors, this simple recipe is for you.

《 Makes 7 cups   Serving size: 1 cup 》

4 qts.	water
1 tbs.	coarse salt
6 oz.	linguine
10 oz.	fresh spinach leaves, stems removed and washed
8 oz.	fresh mushrooms, washed and sliced
6-oz.	jar marinated artichoke hearts, drained and thinly sliced
6	whole peeled canned tomatoes, cut into thin strips
12	large pitted black olives, halved lengthwise
1 tbs.	olive oil
⅛ tsp.	garlic powder or 2 garlic cloves, freshly minced

1. Bring 4 quarts of water to a rolling boil in a large pot. Add salt.
2. Add pasta to boiling water. Stir until all strands are completely submerged.
3. Once water returns to a boil, cook pasta, uncovered, for 8 minutes, stirring occasionally. DO NOT OVER-COOK.
4. While pasta is cooking, place spinach in a strainer and rinse under cold water.
5. Place the spinach in a large frying pan with just the water clinging to its leaves. Cover and cook over medium-high heat for a few minutes until spinach leaves are wilted. Remove from pan, drain, and set aside.

6. Away from the flame, spray the same pan with vegetable spray, add the mushrooms and sauté for 3 minutes.
7. Return the spinach to the pan and add the artichokes, tomatoes, and olives. Mix well.
8. Drizzle olive oil over vegetables and stir.
9. When the pasta is cooked, drain well and add to the vegetables in the pan, sprinkle garlic powder or minced garlic. Mix well. Serve immediately.

EACH SERVING CONTAINS:
173 calories, 29 grams carbohydrate, 6 grams protein, 5 grams fat, 0 milligrams cholesterol, 4 grams fiber

G.I. = LOW

8

GOOD CARBS FOR KIDS

They may sometimes act older than their years, but when it comes to nutritional requirements, *children are not little adults.* Kids have unique caloric and nutritional needs that change as they grow. They also view food differently than adults do: Whether a food is healthful or not has absolutely no bearing on whether they'll eat it. And kids may ignore hunger pangs if they're having more fun playing with a friend or riding their bikes. But food, especially nutrient-dense food, is essential to kids' health and normal development.

Yet as important as diet is to a child's growth, it seems that many kids are missing out on the healthy diets that their bodies require. Here's the proof:

- Thirteen percent of children ages six to eleven years are overweight.
- Fourteen percent of teenagers twelve to nineteen years are overweight.
- Only 2 percent of school-aged children meet the Food Guide Pyramid serving recommendations for all five major food groups.
- About 10 million school-aged children are at health risks due to excess weight.
- About 10 percent of adolescents aged twelve to nineteen have elevated cholesterol.

These numbers reflect the weight status of *American* children. Ongoing research continues to suggest that the prevalence of childhood overweight and obesity is much greater in the U.S. than *anywhere else in the world.* These statistics scream to parents, doctors, teachers, and community and government leaders to *do something* to help our kids! And it's *because children are not little adults that we must help them.*

That All-Important First Year

Infants grow faster during their first year of life than at any other time, so their energy requirements are enormous. A healthy baby's birth weight will double in about the first four months of life and triple by the first year. Babies get the energy and nutrients for this fast growth from their food—breast milk or formula and eventually baby food. Because babies are small, they need small quantities of food. But as the box below clearly shows, based on their body weight, babies need about triple the calories that a grown man needs! And to promote healthy growth, those calories should be nutrient-packed and balanced.

> **Did You Know . . .** that an adult man weighing 175 pounds can meet his nutritional needs by eating 2,400 calories a day? That breaks down to about 14 calories per pound of body weight. But a four-month-old infant weighing 14 pounds needs about 630 calories a day, or about 45 calories per pound of body weight. (If that 175-pound man ate according to an infant's needs, he'd consume close to 8,000 calories every day!)

Babies Need Fat

Infants under two years of age need adequate fat in their diets to grow properly—that's why caregivers should feed these babies whole milk, not low-fat or skim.

Growing Bodies Need More Calories

As babies grow into toddlers, small children, and then school-age children, their energy and nutrient needs naturally grow with them. For example, one-year-old children require about 1,000 calories a day, and by age ten, their energy needs jump to 2,000 calories a day. Parents can best meet their children's energy demands by feeding them a daily diet of nutrient-dense, healthful foods—not a steady diet of *calorie-dense* but *nutrient-empty* foods.

Older Kids—and Food

Adolescents are notorious for eating huge amounts of food. (Boys take the prize for food consumption, though, with their bottomless stomachs!) Children's energy needs are determined by their body size, current growth rate, and physical activity level. Because boys tend to grow faster (once they start) and develop more lean body mass than girls, their energy needs are especially high. Girls usually start to grow earlier than boys and finish their growth spurt sooner too. The growth spurts of average adolescent girls last about five years (from ages ten to fifteen); the same growth spurt in adolescent boys takes about seven years (from ages twelve to nineteen). So girls' high energy needs peak earlier and decline faster than their male peers.

Teenagers can develop horrible eating habits that may haunt them long into their adult years: They may skip meals or eat large pizzas late at night; they may be able to "get away with" eating lots of junk food, and empty-calorie meals and snacks while their bodies are using up so much energy to grow. But once growth levels off and energy requirements drop, where will all those extra empty-calorie calories go? (If you're not sure about the answer, take a look at Chapter 5 and weight control.)

The best way for growing teenagers to meet their daily sky-high nutritional needs is by following the 40-Plus well-balanced diet shown on the Food Pyramid. (See Chapter 1.)

THE FOOD PYRAMID FOR CHILDREN

Fats
Oils
Sweets
(USE SPARINGLY)

Milk, Yogurt, Cheese
2–3 SERVINGS

Meat, Poultry, Fish, Dried Beans, Eggs, Nuts
2–3 SERVINGS

Vegetables
3–4 SERVINGS

Fruits
2–3 SERVINGS

Bread, Cereal, Rice, Pasta
6–9 SERVINGS

Adapted from The Glucose Revolution Pocket Guide to Children with Type 1 Diabetes. Reprinted courtesy of Marlowe & Company.

Better Nutrition for School Children

A bill called Better Nutrition for School Children Act of 2001 has been proposed in the U.S. Senate. If passed, the bill will help address the rise of obesity and type 2 diabetes in children by, among other things, banning the sale of some unhealthful foods (such as soda) on school grounds.

Food: A Kid's Best Friend or Worst Enemy?

Who hasn't seen a young child refuse to eat his peas? Or spinach? Or drink even a small glass of milk? How can a child, you ask yourself, eat macaroni and cheese every single night for dinner and not even consider trying something else? What makes a teenager refuse to bring lunch to school until her best friend starts doing it? There are lots of obstacles that stand in the way of getting good, healthful foods into growing children. Here are a few of them.

Pint-size stomachs. Small children's stomachs fill up fast. So the trick is to get them to eat the most healthful stuff first. That way, they'll get the nutrients they need before getting too full. Little children should be served little portions of a variety of foods; as they grow, food portions should grow along with them.

Picky palates. Children's mouths are very sensitive to temperature, and children also have more taste buds than adults. These differences might explain, then, why children tend to like only a small variety of foods. As they grow, older children usually start liking more diverse flavors, textures, and temperatures. It's a good idea to expose children to a wide variety of foods, though, including vegetables, fruits, and whole-grain breads and cereals; try to make them as interesting and flavorful as possible. Kids don't care about their health or good nutrition; food has to taste good or they won't eat it.

Proof of independence. Children's need to declare their independence can also show up at mealtime. As children mature, these issues begin to fade, especially when parents handle the battles with patience, respect, and understanding.

Peer pressure. All kids want to fit in. And kids will want to eat like their friends and classmates whether in nursery school or college. Unfortunately, the most popular foods are not always the most healthful (in fact, they're almost *never* the most healthful) so this desire to be like everyone else means eating, like everyone else, high-calorie foods with little or no nutritional value. As long as the "junk" foods that children eat at school are offset by healthful meals and snacks at home, there's no real problem. The peer-pressure factor must be given time to run its course.

Now, we can't expect a five-year-old to understand that a daily diet of burgers and fries will, over time, leave plaque deposits on artery walls and possibly lead to a premature heart attack. We know for sure that no teenager looks up the vitamin or mineral content of a food before deciding whether to eat it. But we also know that many young people are teased and suffer real psychological pain because they're overweight. And now more children than ever are being diagnosed with type 2 diabetes—formerly called *adult-onset* diabetes—because of their unhealthful lifestyles.

The Numbers Tell It All

If you do have a hankering for fast food, it's better to avoid the super-sized meals. (One key to a balanced diet is moderation.) For example, compare these numbers:

Regular (moderate) portions	Super-sized portions
McD burger	Big Xtra! with cheese
Small fries	Super-sized fries
16-oz. Coke	Super-sized Coke
627 calories	1,805 calories
19 grams of fat	84 grams of fat

Let's Identify the Problems

Kids need to eat a well-balanced diet of adequate—not excessive—calories and be physically active every day. Nothing new, you say. Not exciting, you say. Well, neither is a child who develops type 2 diabetes in middle school. Or kids not being able to play, run, or bike with kindergarten friends because they're obese. Or young people having heart attacks at twenty-one. Unfortunately, these tragic events are happening to more and more children and young adults every day. What's more, experts tell us that this trend is only going to get worse.

Do things have to get worse? No—not if a few dietary and exercise changes can make the difference. After all, we all have to eat anyway, right? So why not think of food as medicine?

To help zero in on the best ways to improve your child's health, you may ask which is more important, diet (meaning the foods we normally eat) or exercise? If children are tired and overweight, they won't feel very motivated or full of the energy they need to ride a bike or play touch football. So, in this case, getting the energy from food could make all the difference. And if children sit in front of the TV, eating chips or cookies, as the pounds and problems keep adding up, exercise could really turn things around. So good health includes both diet *and* exercise. Let's take a look at the two major causes of young people's expanding waistlines.

Cause #1: Our children overeat. Why? Because in this country, you can get food everywhere, at any hour of any day. And that food is often cheap and high in fats and calories. For example: You pay $4.99 for an Italian hero at a 24-hour convenience store. That one item contains 800 calories and 32 grams of fat!

We live in a culture of portion distortion. If you compare recommendations from the Food Guide Pyramid for daily portions and super-sized meals and snacks, you'll be shocked at the differences. For example, one McDonald's quarter-pounder with cheese, medium fries, and a Coke contains 980 calories, 46 grams fat, 10 teaspoons sugar, and 1,300 mg sodium. That's about 50 percent of the calories, 69 percent of the fat, 80 percent of the sugar, and 57 percent of the sodium that a ten- or twelve-year-old needs *for the whole day*! (And these numbers don't represent super-sized portions.) Try these tips to help your child eat a more balanced diet:

Set a good example. If you want your child to eat a more healthful diet and get more exercise, why not show the way? Prepare meals that are healthful for the whole family and eat them yourself.

Ask your child to help. If you ask them, your kids will help you shop and prepare healthful foods and meals. Have them pick out the apples at the supermarket or prepare the salad for dinner. They're more likely to take pride in (and eat) a meal in which they've been involved.

Cut fruits and vegetables into finger-food sizes. Presenting healthful foods in an interesting way can make them more fun for small children to eat.

Ask your child to help plan the menu. If your child helps you plan menus, he'll pick foods he enjoys (and you can help guide him toward appropriate choices).

Cause #2: Our kids are inactive. Why? Because carpools take our children to and from school and after-school activities, and parents' and kids' tight schedules don't allow a lot of time for scheduled exercise. What's more, kids spend a lot of time watching TV or sitting at the computer instead of playing outside. And kids' poor diets and lack of energy make them too tired, too overweight, or too sick-feeling to run and play. Here are some ways to get your child to become more physically active:

Do things as a family. Why not start some new traditions and go for walks or bike rides as a family? Like to do yard work? Make it a game and ask the kids to help. Not only will you all be getting great exercise, you'll be spending time together too.

Be a role model. If your kids see you gardening, washing the car, raking leaves, and taking evening walks, they'll recognize your good example and be more likely to follow your lead.

Work exercise into every day. Our bodies were built to move, so why not get your child to include more *move*ment throughout the day? After all, walking and climbing stairs don't require special equipment, club memberships, or skills. If you can help make exercise part of your kid's ordinary day, then there's no need to make time for exercise, it's already there.

➤ that 91 percent of food commercials shown during children's programming advertise foods that are either high-fat, high-sugar, or high-salt?

➤ that the American Academy of Pediatrics recommends limiting TV time to a maximum of two hours a day? Research shows that the more a child watches TV, the greater the risk for higher cholesterol levels.

Trickler Carbs to the Rescue

Energy comes from the food we eat. When adults eat a diet of healthful foods that provides consistent amounts of energy throughout the day, they don't feel draggy. In fact, there always seems to be enough energy to keep going. Food works the same way in young bodies. So an energetic child will go to school, participate in some exercise after school (such as soccer, ballet, or swimming), do homework, take part in family chores, and then go to bed—all on the energy that came from that day's breakfast, lunch, dinner, and snacks.

But what *kind* of breakfast, lunch, dinner, and snacks? Nutrient-dense, well-balanced meals and snacks provide the right amount of calories, vitamins, protein, and minerals that growing bodies need to keep going all day long. And low-G.I. carbs included in these meals and snacks assure that steady supply of energy to have—and enjoy—a physically active day.

Trickler carbs work the same in young bodies as they do in older ones. These carbs provide:

◗ Energy that kids need throughout the school day to concentrate and stay mentally alert. A drifting mind sometimes means a hungry body.

▶ A steady supply of energy that carries over to after-school activities. Sometimes, kids show little interest in extracurricular activities because their blood-sugar levels are low.

▶ A feeling of satisfaction or fullness, preventing kids from eating unnecessary calories. Let's face it: Sometimes kids eat because low glucose levels make them *feel* hungry, not because they've actually run out of food calories to burn for energy.

So, to repeat the most healthful diet prescription for a young, growing body:

Eat a well-balanced diet of adequate—not excessive—calories, *including slowly digested carbohydrates* and be physically active every day.

The Ideal Fiber Formula for Kids: An Easy Numbers Game

Can't figure out how much fiber your child should be eating? Try this:

Take your child's age and add five. That gives you the right daily amount of fiber (in grams) the child should be getting. Secret: As children grow, so should their fiber intake.

Example: Five-year-old's fiber needs: 5 + 5 = 10 grams
Six-year-old's fiber needs: 6 + 5 = 11 grams

Before you know it, your child has developed a healthful habit.

Where Do I Find Fiber?

Looking for good fiber sources for your kids? Here are a few:

A slice of whole-grain bread = 2 grams

Medium-sized piece of fruit = 2 grams

Half-cup cooked veggies = 2 grams

Half-cup legumes (such as beans and lentils) = 6 grams

Trickler Carbs and Kids

Question: Why do young people have high nutritional needs?

Answer: Because they're growing.

Question: How can caregivers best meet these high nutritional needs?

Answer: By encouraging kids to eat a well-balanced diet that contains a variety of nutrient-dense foods.

Question: What foods are nutrient-dense but not excessively high in calories, yet provide a steady source of energy to prevent hunger?

Answer: Low-G.I. carbs.

Is Your Child Overweight?

Wondering whether your child is overweight? Here's how to find out: The next time you visit your pediatrician, ask him/her to plot your child's height and weight on a chart. If your child's percentile for weight is much greater than his percentile for height, that's a warning sign. (That may not hold true, though, for boys in early adolescence, who are about to go through their growth spurts. That's when boys build heavy muscles, which can skew the charts.) Also, any child with a BMI greater than the 95th percentile for age and sex is considered overweight.

Bye-Bye, Baby Fat

The old-fashioned view that baby fat melts off by adolescence just doesn't hold true anymore, because today's kids have developed unhealthful eating and lifestyle habits that prevent baby fat from ever melting! And the statistics prove it. Years ago, when baby fat was reserved just for babies, there was no fast food, no eating out, no computers, and no sitting in front of the TV for hours on end. Now these lifestyle habits continue from childhood into adolescence and beyond, so *baby* fat turns into *adult* fat.

Betsy's Story

Betsy, a second-grader, lives with her parents and younger sibling. Betsy is the only person in her family with a weight problem; she weighs 80 pounds and stands just 3'8"; her weight is off the growth chart. For her height, Betsy is considered severely obese. The pediatrician advised Betsy's mother to talk to a registered dietitian for advice; the goal was for Betsy to lose about eight pounds over the next twelve months (the 10% Solution). Betsy's mom thought this was a great idea: She would learn more about healthy eating for her daughter and the entire family.

Betsy's Diet: Before Carb Counseling

Breakfast: Three-quarters cup Rice Chex, 4 oz. 1% milk

Snack: Eight oz. 1% milk, breakfast bar

Lunch: Two ounces turkey breast on small roll, ½ cup instant mashed potatoes with gravy, 8 oz. 1% milk

Snack: Two Oreo cookies, ice cream sandwich

Dinner: A small bowl commercial chicken noodle soup, 5 saltines, cup of orange soda

Snack: Half an orange

Betsy's diet needed lots of changes. For starters, she was eating about 1,700 calories, about 300 more than she needed in a day. And though she drank enough milk to meet the minimal calcium needs of a seven-year-old, on some days she wasn't getting enough high-quality protein foods (from foods such as meat, fish, and eggs). Her fiber intake was low because she ate little fruits, vegetables, and whole grains. Her limited food choices meant that she might not be getting enough vitamins and minerals from her diet. She complained of being too tired to play after school and said she was hungry all the time. Because she was obese at such a young age, Betsy could face weight-related health problems later in life if she doesn't make some changes now.

How Could Betsy Improve Her Diet?

Betsy could start eating better meals by decreasing her starch intake; most of the starches in her diet come from gushers— Rice Chex, instant mashed potatoes, white-flour rolls, cookies, saltines, and soda. For these starches, she could substitute tricklers such as whole-grain cereals, breads, and crackers, and some slowly digested fruits and vegetables. These changes will allow Betsy to eat fewer—yet still enough—calories. What's more, she'll have more energy and feel fuller longer. In the process, she'll be eating balanced meals that meet the demanding nutrient needs of a growing seven-year-old. With her newfound energy, Betsy could look forward to active play time every day after school.

Betsy's Diet: After Carb Counseling

Breakfast: Three-quarters cup Life cereal, 4 oz. 1% milk, $\frac{1}{2}$ cup of strawberries

Snack: Half a sandwich-size bag of green grapes (about 17), 4 oz. 1% milk

Lunch: Ham and reduced-fat-Swiss sandwich, 2 slices rye bread (crusts removed), 6 baby carrots, 4 oz. 1% milk

Snack: A handful of Teddy Grahams, 4 oz. 1% milk

Dinner: Baked chicken drumstick, breaded, without skin, $\frac{1}{3}$ cup mashed sweet potato, $\frac{1}{2}$ cup steamed green beans with vinaigrette, $\frac{1}{2}$ cup of natural applesauce, 4 oz. 1% milk

Snack: Half cup low-fat cooked pudding

Betsy's Back on the Growth Charts

By making small but consistent changes to her diet, Betsy lost seven pounds in eight months. During the end-of-the-year holiday season, her mom thought it would be best to help her maintain that loss, and once the normal school routine started again, work at losing that final pound so that she would reach her goal weight. When Betsy returned to her doctor for her annual physical exam, he was pleased with how well he found her; with her eight-pound loss from the prior year, her weight was back on the growth chart again. The doctor encouraged Betsy and her mom to continue with their current dietary program and check back in six months.

Betsy's mom, thrilled that her little girl has more energy and is less moody, is especially pleased that meal and snack times no longer involve mother-daughter battles.

Tom's Story

Tom discovered that he had elevated blood fats when he was a sophomore in high school and just fifteen and a half years old. He carried 143 pounds on his 5'4" body frame; he was overweight. His doctor was concerned about Tom's frightening cholesterol profile: His bad cholesterol was very high, his good cholesterol was low, and his fasting triglyceride levels were also very high. Because there's a strong history of heart disease and diabetes on both sides of Tom's family, and because adolescents aren't usually treated for high cholesterol with medication, Tom's mom hoped that a better diet would be her son's "pill."

Tom didn't smoke or drink alcohol; he played tennis once or twice a week and forced himself to walk two miles every day since his most recent doctor's visit. He admitted that he was willing to eat a very limited variety of acceptable foods, which included two or three types of fruits and vegetables, no ham, no fish, and no cheese, except on pizza.

Tom's diet (summer schedule): Before Carb Counseling

Breakfast (10:30 a.m.): Three cups Froot Loops, 8 oz. 1% milk
Snack: Eight oz. ginger ale
Lunch: One slice cheese pizza, can Coke
Snack: Eight oz. ginger ale
Dinner: Fried chicken breast (with skin), cucumber and carrot sticks, pickle, 8 oz. ginger ale
Snack: Two or three scoops of sherbet
Snack: An apple, 8 oz. orange juice, 12 oz. 1% chocolate milk

On this kind of a day (and there was little variation in his choices from day to day), Tom consumed about 2,100 calories, which is at the low end of the appropriate range for his daily energy needs. His fat intake (approximately 50 grams) was only about 21 percent of his total calories. But about 40 percent of his total caloric intake came from nutritional "lightweights" such as Froot Loops, soda, and sherbet. These foods gave his body empty calories; that is, his body did all the work of breaking them down into glucose but that's all he got—just glucose, not very many of the 40-Plus nutrients he also needed. His diet lacked fiber and heart-healthful fats and contained a lot of hidden sugar (probably between forty-five and fifty teaspoons!). No wonder he complained of being tired and hungry all the time, didn't feel like playing sports or being physically active during his summer vacation. Tom was on a daily roller-coaster ride of blood-sugar highs and lows.

How Could Tom Improve His Diet?

Wow! Forty-five to fifty teaspoons of sugar in a day gave Tom a *long* roller-coaster ride too. His weight gain and high triglyceride levels were no surprise, given the way he was eating and his family's medical history. By agreeing to eat whole-grain cereals and breads, and including more fruits and vegetables throughout the day, Tom would quickly feel more energetic all day long. He would also lose weight gradually, because low-G.I. foods help you burn fat more readily rather than store it. (See Chapter 4 for a detailed explanation). Perhaps most important of all, a low-G.I. diet would help Tom attack his elevated cholesterol and triglycerides.

Tom's Diet: After Carb Counseling

Breakfast: One and a half cups 100% Bran Flakes, 8 oz. skim Plus milk, water with a multivitamin pill

Lunch: Sandwich (turkey, chicken, or fat-free bologna), 2 slices rye bread, cucumber spears, apple, water *or* (on days when he worked at the pizza shop): slice cheese pizza, apple, diet Coke

Dinner: One or two ears corn, grilled chicken breast (no skin), broccoli with olive oil (he loves the way his mom makes this and eats 2 cups), 2 handfuls grapes, water

Snack: Twelve oz. 1% chocolate milk, 2 to 3 fat-free oatmeal cookies

Tom's Energy Surge

Although his new diet plan wasn't ideal, it was a huge improvement. Most important, Tom agreed that he could live with it. After six months of his new lifestyle, Tom's cholesterol dropped 136 points, putting him well within the normal range. The same was true for his LDL (bad) cholesterol, which dropped

98 points; his fasting triglycerides also fell 184 points. In other words, all of his blood values that used to be out of the normal range were now back to normal. Tom lost 19 pounds; he ate fewer *empty* calories, although he was still eating about the same *number* of calories. He also got more exercise (he swam and went bike riding most days). And because he had more energy, he didn't have to force himself into activity. His doctor was amazed at Tom's new blood levels and his mother was relieved that she now had a plan to help her son eat better and improve his health. And Tom was happy that everyone was off his case. He says: "I know I'm still a picky eater, but I think I've done great, and even better, so does my mother!"

THE BOTTOM LINE

➤ Children's nutritional needs are not the same as those of adults.

➤ Kids have unique caloric and nutrient needs that change as they grow.

➤ Infants grow faster during their first year of life than at any other time.

➤ Infants under two years of age need adequate fat in their diet to grow properly.

➤ Like adults, children and young people should eat a well-balanced diet of adequate—not excessive—calories, *including slowly digested carbohydrates* and be physically active every day.

Smashed Sweet
Potato-Carrot Puree

DON'T save this recipe just for Thanksgiving dinner. Why not give your body the vitamin A, potassium, and fiber contained in both the sweet potatoes and carrots throughout the year—and delight your taste buds at the same time?

❨ **Makes 4½ cups   Serving size: ½ cup** ❩

2 lbs.	sweet potatoes or yams, scrubbed, ends cut off
1 lb.	baby carrots
2 cups	water
1 tbs.	brown sugar
3 tbs.	butter or margarine
	salt and pepper to taste
½ cup	light sour cream
½ tsp.	nutmeg
1 tbs.	cognac or port or sherry wine

1. Bake, steam, or microwave potatoes until tender. (Time will depend on size of potato and cooking method; the longest cooking time: baked for one hour at 375°.)
2. Place carrots in medium saucepan with 2 cups water, brown sugar, butter or margarine, salt and pepper. Cook, uncovered, over medium heat about 30 minutes or until tender, making sure all water has evaporated. When cooked, place in the bowl of a food processor fitted with a steel blade.
3. When sweet potatoes are cooked, cool for easy handling. Scrape out the flesh with a spoon and add potatoes to carrots in the processor.

4. Combine sour cream, nutmeg, and cognac or wine. Add to vegetables and process until very smooth.
5. Taste to correct seasonings.
6. Transfer puree to 9-inch-square baking dish, cover, and heat thoroughly in an oven preheated to 350°.
7. Serve steaming hot.

EACH SERVING CONTAINS:
130 calories, 20 grams carbohydrate, 2 grams protein, 5 grams fat, 14 milligrams cholesterol, 3 grams fiber

G.I. = LOW

9

GOOD CARBS
FOR PEAK PERFORMANCE

Whether you're sleeping, thinking, eating, singing, or running a marathon, glucose makes you move. And there's a specific relationship between your movements and the source of the energy (carbs) that fuels those movements.

If you look at the parking lot outside an office building or shopping mall, you'll see lots of cars of all different sizes and shapes, makes and colors, capabilities and prices. But they all share one thing in common: They all need fuel to move. And not just any fuel will work in these vehicles. Cars need the fuel they were built to run on—gasoline.

Your body, just like a car, runs on its own preferred fuel—glucose. And the best "pump" from which to get this fuel is dietary carbs. Your body has an easier time extracting energy from carbs than it does from fats or proteins, the other foods you eat.

So when you're thinking about different energy sources for exercise, it's important to know that your body prefers carbs. Because carbohydrates are your body's fuel of choice, it doesn't have to work as hard to get energy. That means that you get lots of energy, although your system has had to do little work. And if your body uses a minimal number of calories to break down its energy source (through carb digestion), there will be more calories left to burn during exercise. That extra energy could mean the difference between finishing the race and *winning* the race!

From the "Sad but True" File

> ➤ Only 22 percent of U.S. adults get the recommended regular physical activity (5 times a week for at least 30 minutes) of any intensity during their leisure time.

> ➤ About 15 percent get the recommended amount of vigorous activity (three times a week for at least 20 minutes).

> ➤ About 25 percent of adults claim they do no physical activity at all in their leisure time.

> ➤ Approximately 25 percent of young people (ages twelve to twenty-one) report getting no vigorous physical activity.

> ➤ Sixty percent of Americans are not regularly active.

> ➤ Just 19 percent of all high school students are physically active for 20 minutes or more in daily physical education classes.

High Test, High Payback

It may be more costly in the short term, but putting high-test gasoline in your car has definite advantages. When you give your car top-notch fuel, it responds with top-notch performance: no knocks or pings, just a dependable, smooth ride every time. Your car will likely spend less time in the repair shop too. Over the years, your car will continue to perform reliably and give you few headaches. *But to perform its best, you need to give it the right kind of fuel.*

Likewise, if you give your system the best fuel possible, it, too, will respond with high performance; it may be high performance in school, at work, or at home; it may be high performance during a basketball game, a race, or an intense workout at the gym. It should come as no surprise to you that the best sources for your glucose fuel are the carbohydrate foods you eat. Let's review why:

▶ Your body digests the food you eat to get the energy contained in those foods. That energy enables you to do absolutely everything—from breathing to recovering from a cold to whistling to white-water rafting.

▶ Just as gasoline makes cars run, glucose makes your system run.

▶ Your system can extract glucose from all types of food, but carbs are the easiest for it to use, since glucose is *already* a carb.

▶ How do carbs benefit you during exercise? By leaving you lots of leftover energy after digestion. That means you have more energy to use for exercise.

It all makes sense, doesn't it? Your body is a machine—just like your car.

Don't Forget Your Water!

You need four to eight ounces of water every fifteen to twenty minutes while you exercise—*whether you're thirsty or not.* This amount is in addition to the eight to twelve cups of water you should already be drinking every day. But no need to worry: All of the beverages you drink contain water, as do most foods you eat, even foods such as bread, nuts, meat, and cheese; the only foods that don't contain water are vegetable oils. By the way, alcohol and caffeinated beverages aren't good fluid sources; they can lead to dehydration.

Trickler Carbs, Your High-Test Fuel

If you can shift your system into "cruise control," you'll find that your energy will last longer, with plenty of time before the "empty" light starts to flash. Quickly digested carbs, gushers, rapidly release just-digested energy into your bloodstream, where insulin quickly responds and hurries it to the cells, leaving you with an exhausted energy supply. So if you're starting to exercise, where will your energy come from if your tank is empty before you even start your trip? In contrast, slowly digested tricklers help you go the distance simply because they drip (or trickle) energy into your blood over a long period of time.

Gushers Aren't All Bad

There are certain circumstances when you need gushers; for example: during prolonged exercise, when you don't want your blood-sugar levels to drop too low, and after intense exercise, when you want to speed up glycogen storage, since you used some glycogen during exercise. (Glycogen, you may remember, is your system's quickly available form of stored energy.)

Tony's Story

Tony, a bachelor in his mid-twenties, works as a full-time fire-fighter, and takes college courses a few nights a week. At 5'9" and 189 pounds (BMI of 28), Tony is overweight. (His goal weight is 170 pounds—the 10% Solution.) Tony has been a serious athlete ever since high school and competes in bi- and triathlons several times a season.

Tony noticed that his performance level had been slipping over the past few competitions and thought that his steady weight gain since high school was part of the problem. He wasn't quite sure how to fix things: He was committed to an intense workout most days, so he knew he was burning lots of calories; but he was also intensely hungry *all* the time—whether he worked out or not. Could he be overeating, with all the regular exercise he was getting?

Tony's family suffered from a strong history of diabetes, heart disease, and obesity, but Tony thought he was insuring himself against these possible health concerns by getting lots of exercise.

Tony's Workout Schedule

Tony keeps to a pretty rigorous training program: Not only does he run a 13-minute mile four to six times a week, he also bikes three times a week for 90 minutes and weight-trains five to seven times a week for 30 minutes.

Tony's Diet: Before Carb Counseling

Breakfast: Two or 3 cups Rice Chex, 16 oz. 2% milk

Snack: Banana, pear, 2 carrots

Lunch: Two slices white sandwich bread, 3 oz. roast beef, 2 handfuls pretzels, 1 cup strawberries, 32 oz. Gatorade

Dinner: One lb. steak, 1½ cups green beans with approx. 2 tbs. butter, 2 cups linguine, 1 cup cream sauce, 32 oz. Gatorade

Late-night snack: One sleeve saltines, 32 oz. Gatorade

Even though Tony stuck to an intense workout schedule, he was eating way too many calories. On an average day, such as the one above, Tony's food intake could add up to about 5,500 calories and over 200 grams of fat! Even for an athlete, this diet resulted in weight gain—as body fat. And given his family's medical history, Tony's diet was placing him in danger of heart disease and possibly diabetes. Reducing his caloric intake by 50 percent would still meet his daily metabolic requirements and give him the energy he needed for his workouts.

How Could Tony Improve His Diet?

Tony would feel fuller longer if he ate a low-G.I. cereal in the morning such as Bran Buds or old-fashioned oatmeal instead of Rice Chex. He could also replace his gusher white bread with a whole-wheat pita or whole-grain pumpernickel bread. Then he could reduce his food portions at other meals throughout the day. His snacks could consist of light yogurt or low-fat milk, oatmeal, or Social Tea biscuits or some ice cream, or chips and salsa. And the only time he should drink 32 ounces of Gatorade, a quickly digested sugar drink, is on those three days a week when he went on a ninety-minute bike ride. For that long bike ride, Tony might need a handy energy source to replenish his body's emptied glucose and glycogen stores.

Tony's Diet: After Carb Counseling

Breakfast: Two cups oat bran cereal, 12 oz. 1% milk, large apple, water

Snack: One to 2 handfuls of grapes

Lunch: Two slices whole-grain pumpernickel, 3 oz. lean roast beef, 1 tbs. mayonnaise, sandwich-sized zip-loc Baggie of raw vegetables (baby carrots, celery, pepper strips), large pear, 2 oatmeal cookies, water

Snack: Low-fat granola bar, 8 oz. 1% milk

Dinner: One and a half cups long-grain rice pilaf, 6 oz. rosemary chicken breast, 2 cups steamed broccoli florets with 2 pats butter and 2 tbs. slivered almonds, water

Snack: Small apple cinnamon muffin (from mix), 8 oz. 1% milk

As you can see, fewer calories don't leave Tony with an empty plate! Yet his new meal plan adds up to 50 percent fewer calories and 70 percent less fat than his old diet. And his meals aren't low-calorie or low-fat; they're just not excessive as they once were.

Tony's New Competitive Edge

In the first five weeks of his new way of eating, Tony dropped seven and a half pounds. Then, after ten weeks, he reached his goal of 170 pounds. In his first competition at his new weight, a biathlon, he finished 66th out of 200-plus competitors, his personal best. Tony says, "I never dreamed I could run so fast or bike so long on half the calories I was used to eating!"

Four years have passed since Tony first began incorporating low-G.I. carbs into his meal and snack planning, and he's still an elite athlete maintaining a healthy weight of 171 pounds. To date, his annual physicals and blood work show no signs of any looming health problems—the best part of this success story.

Reaching the Finish Line

Low-G.I. carbohydrates provide you with a slow, steady flow of energy that lasts for a prolonged period of time. What's more, these foods don't cause sugar highs and lows; tricklers offer no roller-coaster rides—just smooth, consistent rides in cruise control.

Whether it's for peak performance or just to improve a workout or physical skill (such as playing tennis or skiing), training is an essential part of exercise: Practice makes perfect. But better fueling is just as crucial. In fact, for some people—Tony's a great example—it may just provide that elusive competitive edge.

THE BOTTOM LINE

➤ Your system, just like a car, "runs" on its own preferred fuel— glucose. The best fuels are dietary carbs.

➤ Your body has an easier time extracting energy from carbs than it does from fats or proteins. That leaves you with more leftover energy for exercise.

➤ Gusher foods come in handy when you don't want your blood-sugar levels to drop too low and when you want to speed up glycogen storage.

➤ Low-G.I. carbohydrates provide you with a slow, steady flow of energy for a prolonged period of time.

➤ Make sure you drink enough fluids throughout the day.

High-Test Granola

MAKE this recipe just once, taste it just once, and store-bought granola will be wiped off your shopping list forever!

❰ **Makes 9 cups   Serving size: ½ cup** ❱

	Vegetable spray
½ cup	honey
6 cups	old-fashioned oats (not quick oats)
1 tbs.	cinnamon
¼ cup	ground flaxseed
¾ cup	slivered almonds (or any other nut, such as pecans, cashews, almonds, or walnuts)
¼ cup	soy nuts
1 cup	dried blueberries and currants (or any other combination of dried fruit, except dates)

1. Spray large baking pan ($9 \times 10 \times 2\frac{1}{2}$) with cooking spray. Add honey.
2. Place pan in cold oven. Turn on oven to 350°.
3. In large bowl, combine next 5 ingredients (oats through soy nuts). Mix well.
4. When honey has melted, remove pan from oven. Add oat mixture to baking pan. Spread and turn to coat well with honey.
5. Bake for 25 minutes or until oats are well toasted, turning every 5 to 6 minutes.
6. Remove from oven. Cool thoroughly.
7. Add dried fruit.
8. Store in airtight container.

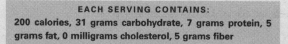

EACH SERVING CONTAINS:
200 calories, 31 grams carbohydrate, 7 grams protein, 5 grams fat, 0 milligrams cholesterol, 5 grams fiber

G.I. = LOW

10

CHOOSE THE RIGHT CARBS
FOR YOU

If there's a message to take home from this book, it's that you should eat a balanced diet that consists of a variety of high-fiber, slowly digested carbohydrates, and heart-healthful proteins and fats. Okay, so how do you transfer this information from your head and onto your plate or into a brown bag? And how can you recognize the best choices on a menu or supermarket shelf?

Maybe the following lists will help: We've provided three breakfast, lunch, and dinner examples, along with a wide variety of snacks. The average nutrient breakdown for these meals (excluding snacks) is 54 percent carbohydrate, 22 percent protein, and 24 percent fat.

Please keep this in mind: The portions of some foods (such as sandwich fillings, pasta, and chicken) may seem small, while other serving sizes (such as those for vegetables and fruits) may seem large. All of the portion sizes that we suggest reflect the Food Guide Pyramid recommendations.

We hope these examples begin to dispel current notions of "portion distortion." As you replace empty-calorie foods with tricklers, fiber, and heart-healthy foods, you'll be amazed at how *so little* (smaller portions and fewer calories) can go *so far* (your energy level). Try not to eat with your eyes, but with your head—a wonderful surprise awaits you!

1,200 daily calories	1,500 daily calories	1,800 daily calories	2,000 daily calories	2,400 daily calories

Ideal calorie range for:

➤ Preadolescent children
➤ Most women who want to lose weight
➤ Inactive adults of small stature

Ideal calorie range for:

➤ Most preteen adolescents
➤ Active women

➤ Older men
➤ Most men who want to lose weight

Ideal calorie range for:

➤ Active teenagers
➤ Large-stature active women
➤ Healthy-weight adult men

Quick-Muffin Breakfast

Fiber-High Bran Muffin*
1 tbs. peanut butter
8 oz. no-sugar-added hot chocolate or 8 oz. skim or 1% milk

Fiber-High Bran Muffin*
1/2 tbs. light margarine
1/2 cup unsweetened canned fruit cocktail
8 oz. no-sugar-added hot chocolate or 8 oz. skim or 1% milk

Fiber-High Bran Muffin*
1 tbs. light cream cheese
Large piece seasonal fruit or 2 cups sliced strawberries
8 oz. no-sugar-added hot chocolate or 8 oz. skim or 1% milk

2 Fiber-High Bran Muffins*
1 tbs. apple butter
1 tbs. light margarine
Large piece seasonal fruit or 2 cups sliced strawberries
8 oz. no-sugar-added hot chocolate or 8 oz. skim or 1% milk

Fiber-High Bran Muffin*
1 tbs. apple butter
2 slices rye or 100% whole wheat toast
2 oz. low-salt boiled ham or reduced-fat cheese
Large piece seasonal fruit or 2 cups sliced strawberries
8 oz. no-sugar-added hot chocolate or 8 oz. skim or 1% milk

*Recipe appears on page 74.

1,200 daily calories	1,500 daily calories	1,800 daily calories	2,000 daily calories	2,400 daily calories

Super Cereal Breakfast

1,200 daily calories	1,500 daily calories	1,800 daily calories	2,000 daily calories	2,400 daily calories
1⅓ cups Special K 6 oz. skim or 1% milk 1 cup unsweetened canned peaches or 1 cup grapes	1⅓ cups Special K 8 oz. skim or 1% milk 1 cup unsweetened canned peaches or 1 cup grapes	1½ cups Special K 8 oz. skim or 1% milk 1 cup unsweetened canned peaches or 1 cup grapes Quaker chewy granola bar or 2 low-fat graham crackers (2 full sheets)	2 cups Special K 16 oz. skim or 1% milk 2 cups unsweetened canned peaches or 2 cups grapes Quaker chewy granola bar or 2 low-fat graham crackers (2 full sheets)	2 cups Special K 16 oz. skim or 1% milk 1 cup unsweetened canned peaches or 1 cup grapes 2 Quaker chewy granola bars or 4 low-fat graham crackers (4 full sheets)

Cooked Cereal Breakfast

1,200 daily calories	1,500 daily calories	1,800 daily calories	2,000 daily calories	2,400 daily calories
½ cup uncooked old-fashioned oats made with water ½ cup Simply Delicious Applesauce* or 1 cup unsweetened canned peaches	½ cup uncooked old-fashioned oats made with water ½ cup Simply Delicious Applesauce* or 1 cup unsweetened canned peaches 4 oz. light yogurt	½ cup uncooked old-fashioned oats made with 1 cup skim or 1% milk ½ cup Simply Delicious Applesauce* or 1 cup unsweetened canned peaches 1 low-fat graham cracker (1 full sheet)	½ cup uncooked old-fashioned oats made with 1 cup skim or 1% milk ½ cup Simply Delicious Applesauce* or 1 cup unsweetened canned peaches 1 sourdough or whole-wheat English muffin 1 tbs. natural, no-salt-added peanut butter 2 tsp. all-fruit spread	¾ cup uncooked old-fashioned oats made with 1½ cups skim or 1% milk ½ cup Simply Delicious Applesauce* or 1 cup unsweetened canned peaches 1 sourdough or whole-wheat English muffin 2 tsp. natural, no-salt-added peanut butter 2 tsp. all-fruit spread

Recipe appears on page 149.

1,200 daily calories	1,500 daily calories	1,800 daily calories	2,000 daily calories	2,400 daily calories

Delicious Deli Lunch

1,200 daily calories	1,500 daily calories	1,800 daily calories	2,000 daily calories	2,400 daily calories
2 slices rye bread	2 slices rye bread	2 slices rye bread	2 slices rye bread	2 slices rye bread
1 oz. turkey breast	1 oz. turkey breast	1 oz. turkey breast	2 oz. turkey breast	2 oz. turkey breast
1 oz. low-fat cheese	1 oz. low-fat cheese	1 oz. low-fat cheese	2 oz. low-fat cheese	2 oz. low-fat cheese
Lettuce	Lettuce	Lettuce	Lettuce	Lettuce
Tomato	Tomato	Tomato	Tomato	Tomato
1 cup cantaloupe or 1 orange	1 cup cantaloupe or 1 orange	1 cup cantaloupe or 1 orange	1½ cups cantaloupe or 1 medium apple	1 tbs. light mayonnaise
4 oz. light yogurt	8 oz. light yogurt	8 oz. light yogurt	8 oz. light yogurt	2 cups cantaloupe or 2 cups grapes
				8 oz. light yogurt
				Quaker chewy granola bar

Wrap Lunch

1,200 daily calories	1,500 daily calories	1,800 daily calories	2,000 daily calories	2,400 daily calories
Goat Cheese Wrap*	Goat Cheese Wrap*	Goat Cheese Wrap*	Goat Cheese Wrap*	2 Goat Cheese Wraps*
1 cup lettuce, tomato, cucumber, and red onion salad	1 cup lettuce, tomato, cucumber, and red onion salad	1 cup lettuce, tomato, cucumber, and red onion salad	1 cup lettuce, tomato, cucumber, and red onion salad	1 cup lettuce, tomato, cucumber, and red onion salad
2 tbs. Good Seasons fat-free dressing	2 tbs. Good Seasons fat-free dressing	2 tbs. Good Seasons fat-free dressing	2 tbs. Good Seasons fat-free dressing	2 tbs. Good Seasons fat-free dressing
4 Pringles Right crisps (⅓ less fat)	8 Pringles Right crisps (⅓ less fat)	8 Pringles Right crisps (⅓ less fat)	8 Pringles Right crisps (⅓ less fat)	1 kiwi or 1 cup strawberries
			2 kiwis or 2 cups strawberries	

*Recipe appears on page 31.

1,200 daily calories	1,500 daily calories	1,800 daily calories	2,000 daily calories	2,400 daily calories

Salad Bar Lunch

1,200 daily calories	1,500 daily calories	1,800 daily calories	2,000 daily calories	2,400 daily calories
1 cup lettuce	1 cup lettuce	1 cup lettuce	1 cup lettuce	1 cup lettuce
2 cups mixed raw vegetables	2 cups mixed raw vegetables	2 cups mixed raw vegetables	2 cups mixed raw vegetables	2 cups mixed raw vegetables
½ cup kidney beans	½ cup kidney beans	½ cup kidney beans	½ cup kidney beans	½ cup kidney beans
¼ cup reduced-fat salad dressing	¼ cup reduced-fat salad dressing	¼ cup reduced-fat salad dressing	¼ cup reduced-fat salad dressing	1 hard-boiled egg
2 Ry-Krisp crackers	3 Ry-Krisp crackers	3 Ry-Krisp crackers	3 Ry-Krisp crackers	¼ cup reduced-fat salad dressing
10 Teddy Grahams	1 oatmeal cookie	1 oatmeal cookie	1 oatmeal cookie	3 Ry-Krisp crackers
			1 medium pear or 8 oz. canned unsweetened pears	2 oatmeal cookies
				1 medium pear or 8 oz. canned, unsweetened pears

Pasta Dinner

1,200 daily calories	1,500 daily calories	1,800 daily calories	2,000 daily calories	2,400 daily calories
1 cup Just-Plain-Good Pasta*	1½ cup Just-Plain-Good Pasta*	1½ cup Just-Plain-Good Pasta*	1½ cup Just-Plain-Good Pasta*	2 cups Just-Plain-Good Pasta*
3 oz. chicken breast, skinless, grilled	3 oz. chicken breast, skinless, grilled	3 oz. chicken breast, skinless, grilled	6 oz. chicken breast, skinless, grilled	6 oz. chicken breast, skinless, grilled
6 asparagus spears, steamed or grilled	9 asparagus spears, steamed or grilled	9 asparagus spears, steamed or grilled	9 asparagus spears, steamed or grilled	12 asparagus spears, steamed or grilled
1 tsp. olive oil or ½ tbs. light whipped margarine	1 tsp. olive oil or ½ tbs. light whipped margarine	1 tsp. olive oil or ½ tbs. light whipped margarine	1 tsp. olive oil or ½ tbs. light whipped margarine	1 tsp. olive oil or ½ tbs. light whipped margarine
½ cup cooked, sugar-free pudding	½ cup cooked, sugar-free pudding	½ cup cooked, sugar-free pudding	Small baked apple or 1 cup sliced strawberries	Small baked apple or 1 cup sliced strawberries
1 tbs. Cool Whip Lite or Dream Whip	1 tbs. Cool Whip Lite or Dream Whip	1 tbs. Cool Whip Lite or Dream Whip	1 tbs. whipped topping	1 tbs. whipped topping

*Recipe appears on page 111.

1,200 daily calories	1,500 daily calories	1,800 daily calories	2,000 daily calories	2,400 daily calories

Fish Dinner

1,200 daily calories	1,500 daily calories	1,800 daily calories	2,000 daily calories	2,400 daily calories
½ cup Saffron Rice Pilaf*	¾ cup Saffron Rice Pilaf*	¾ cup Saffron Rice Pilaf*	1 cup Saffron Rice Pilaf*	1 cup Saffron Rice Pilaf*
3 oz. salmon, grilled or poached, or 6 oz. cod, broiled	4 oz. salmon, grilled or poached, or 8 oz. cod, broiled	4 oz. salmon, grilled or poached, or 8 oz. cod, broiled	4 oz. salmon, grilled or poached, or 8 oz. cod, broiled	5 oz. salmon, grilled or poached, or 10 oz. cod, broiled
1½ cups or 2 stalks broccoli, steamed	1 cup or 1 stalk broccoli, steamed	1 cup or 1 stalk broccoli, steamed	1 cup or 1 stalk broccoli, steamed	1½ cups or 2 stalks broccoli, steamed
2 tsp. olive oil or 1 tbs. light whipped margarine	2 tsp. olive oil or 1 tbs. light whipped margarine	2 tsp. olive oil or 1 tbs. light whipped margarine	2 tsp. olive oil or 1 tbs. light whipped margarine	2 tsp. olive oil or 1 tbs. light whipped margarine
1 cup citrus sections or 1½ cups fresh fruit salad	1 cup citrus sections or 1½ cups fresh fruit salad	1 cup citrus sections or 1½ cups fresh fruit salad	1 cup citrus sections or 1½ cups fresh fruit salad	1 cup citrus sections or 1½ cups fresh fruit salad

*Recipe appears on page 90.

Meatless Dinner

1,200 daily calories	1,500 daily calories	1,800 daily calories	2,000 daily calories	2,400 daily calories
1 cup So-Sweet Pepper Soup*	1 cup So-Sweet Pepper Soup*	1 cup So-Sweet Pepper Soup*	1½ cups So-Sweet Pepper Soup*	1½ cups So-Sweet Pepper Soup*
2-egg mushroom omelet	2-egg mushroom omelet	2-egg mushroom omelet	2-egg mushroom omelet	2-egg and 1-oz. low-fat cheddar-mushroom omelet
Mini-pita, toasted	2-oz. pita, toasted	2-oz. pita, toasted	2-oz. pita, toasted	2-oz. pita, toasted
1 cup steamed green beans or spinach	1 cup steamed green beans or spinach	1 cup steamed green beans or spinach	1 cup steamed green beans or spinach	2 cups steamed green beans or spinach
1 tsp. olive oil	1 tsp. olive oil	1 tsp. olive oil	2 tsp. olive oil	2 tsp. olive oil
2 fresh apricots or ¾ cup sliced strawberries	4 fresh apricots or 1½ cups sliced strawberries	4 fresh apricots or 1½ cups sliced strawberries	4 fresh apricots or 1½ cups sliced strawberries	4 fresh apricots or 1½ cups sliced strawberries

*Recipe appears on page 12.

The Snack Shack

You'll notice that we've listed a certain number of snack calories for every calorie plan below. So no matter which meal plan you choose, it's okay to eat snacks. For example, the 1,200-calorie meal allows you to add in 100 snack calories. And if your meal plan calls for a 200-calorie snack, you'll want to include two 100-calorie snacks or one 200-calorie snack, and so on.

1,200 daily calories: Add in 100 snack calories
1,500 daily calories: Add in 200 snack calories
1,800 daily calories: Add in 400 snack calories
2,000 daily calories: Add in 200 snack calories
2,400 daily calories: Add in 300 snack calories

Here are some trickler snacks that will keep you feeling satisfied no matter how many calories you're eating.

100-Calorie Snacks

❱ 1 Quaker chewy granola bar
❱ 18 Teddy Grahams
❱ 1½ graham-cracker sheets
❱ 11 sourdough pretzel nuggets
❱ 28 pistachios
❱ 8 walnut halves
❱ 22 dry-roasted peanuts
❱ 29 cherries
❱ 1¼ cups blueberries
❱ 1¾ cups grapes
❱ 8 oz. skim or 1% milk
❱ 6–8 oz. light yogurt
❱ 1 pear
❱ 1½ cups honeydew

❱ 17 small baked tortilla chips and ¼ cup refrigerated salsa

❱ ½ cup soft-serve frozen yogurt

❱ ½ cup ice milk

❱ ⅛ slice avocado and 3 Ry-Krisp crackers

❱ 1 oz. part-skim mozzarella and 1 Wasa bread

200-Calorie Snacks

❱ 2 low-fat oatmeal cookies

❱ 1 Fiber-High Bran Muffin* and 1 tbs. all-fruit jelly

❱ 6 Lorna Doone cookies

❱ ¼ cup soy nuts

❱ 26 almonds

❱ 1 cup Simply Delicious Applesauce**

❱ 7 dried peach halves

❱ ¾ cup Healthy Choice ice cream

❱ 6 to 8 oz. light yogurt and ¼ cup High-Test Granola***

❱ 12 oz. skim or 1% milk and 2 tbs. Lite Hershey chocolate syrup

❱ 6 stoneground wheat crackers and 2 tbs. hummus

❱ 1 fruit smoothie (8 oz. skim or 1% milk and 1½–2 cups berries)

*Recipe appears on page 74.

**Recipe appears on page 149

***Recipe appears on page 139.

To Wrap Up

Experience tells you that if you keep doing the same things in the same ways, you'll keep getting the same results. So why not try something new? If you're looking to make positive changes to improve your health and boost your energy, we hope that you'll try some of our recommendations. Over time, these healthful changes will become habits and simply part of your new, healthful lifestyle.

Now you know what your body has known all along— **carbohydrates rule!**

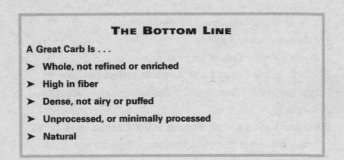

THE BOTTOM LINE

A Great Carb Is . . .

➤ Whole, not refined or enriched

➤ High in fiber

➤ Dense, not airy or puffed

➤ Unprocessed, or minimally processed

➤ Natural

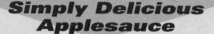

Simply Delicious Applesauce

Here's a perfect example in cooking when less is *definitely* better. The only simpler way to eat an apple is straight off the tree!

❪ **Makes 5 ½ cups   Serving size: ½ cup** ❫

4 lbs.	mixed apples (Gala, Macintosh, Rome Beauty, Cortland)
1 tbs.	vanilla extract
1 tsp.	cinnamon

1. Core and peel apples. Slice into eighths and then cut in half horizontally.
2. Place apple chunks into a wide-based pot and cover. Do not add water.
3. Cook over medium-low heat for approximately 30 minutes or until mixture reaches desired consistency. Stir every few minutes to prevent sticking.
4. Remove apples from heat.
5. Add in vanilla and cinnamon and mix thoroughly.
6. May be served warm or cold.
7. Store in refrigerator.

> **EACH SERVING CONTAINS:**
> 95 calories, 23 grams carbohydrate, less than 1 gram protein, less than 1 gram fat, 0 milligrams cholesterol, 3 grams fiber
>
> G.I. = LOW

APPENDIX:
THE GLYCEMIC INDEX VALUES
OF SOME POPULAR FOODS

As you look over the list on the following pages, notice that the food categories are limited to starch, simple sugar, fruit, and dairy—all types of carbs. And keep in mind that we classify a food's Glycemic Index this way:

Gusher foods	High G.I. (greater than 70)
Intermediate foods	G.I. of 55–70
Trickler foods	Low G.I. (less than 55)

Food	G.I. Level	Food Category
A		
Angel food cake	Intermediate	Starch
Apple juice, unsweetened	Trickler	Fruit
Apple	Trickler	Fruit
Apple, dried	Trickler	Fruit
Apricot jam, no added sugar	Intermediate	Fruit
Apricots, canned, light syrup	Intermediate	Fruit
Apricots		
dried	Trickler	Fruit
fresh	Intermediate	Fruit
Arrowroot	Intermediate	Starch
B		
Bagel	Gusher	Starch
Baked beans	Trickler	Starch
Banana bread	Trickler	Starch
Banana, raw	Intermediate	Fruit
Barley, pearl, boiled	Trickler	Starch
Beets, canned, drained	Intermediate	Vegetable
Black bean soup	Intermediate	Starch
Black beans, boiled	Trickler	Starch
Black-eyed peas, canned	Trickler	Starch
Bread stuffing from mix	Gusher	Starch
Breads		
Kaiser roll	Gusher	Starch
100% stoneground whole-wheat	Trickler	Starch
dark rye, black bread	Gusher	Starch
dark rye, Schinkenbröt	Gusher	Starch
French baguette	Gusher	Starch
hamburger bun	Intermediate	Starch
light deli (American) rye	Intermediate	Starch
Melba toast	Intermediate	Starch
pita bread, whole-wheat	Intermediate	Starch
pumpernickel, whole-grain	Trickler	Starch

Food	G.I. Level	Food Category
rye	Intermediate	Starch
sourdough rye, Arnold's	Intermediate	Starch
sourdough	Trickler	Starch
white	Gusher	Starch
whole-wheat	Intermediate	Starch
Breakfast cereals		
All-Bran with Extra Fiber, Kellogg's	Trickler	Starch
Bran Buds with Psyllium, Kellogg's	Trickler	Starch
Bran Flakes, Post	Gusher	Starch
Cheerios, General Mills	Gusher	Starch
Cocoa Krispies, Kellogg's	Gusher	Starch
Corn Bran, Quaker Crunchy	Gusher	Starch
Corn Chex	Gusher	Starch
Corn Flakes, Kellogg's	Gusher	Starch
Cream of Wheat, instant	Gusher	Starch
Cream of Wheat, old fashioned, cooked	Intermediate	Starch
Crispix, Kellogg's	Gusher	Starch
Frosted Flakes, Kellogg's	Intermediate	Starch
Golden Grahams, General Mills	Gusher	Starch
Grapenuts Flakes, Post	Gusher	Starch
Grapenuts, Post	Intermediate	Starch
Just Right	Intermediate	Starch
Life, Quaker	Intermediate	Starch
Mini Wheats (whole-wheat)	Intermediate	Starch
Muesli, toasted	Trickler	Starch
Muesli, natural muesli	Intermediate	Starch
Multi-Bran Chex, General Mills	Intermediate	Starch
Oat bran, Quaker Oats	Trickler	Starch
Oatmeal (made with water), old-fashioned, cooked	Trickler	Starch

Food	G.I. Level	Food Category
Oats, 1-minute, Quaker	Intermediate	Starch
Puffed Wheat, Quaker	Intermediate	Starch
Raisin Bran, Kellogg's	Gusher	Starch
Rice Chex, General Mills	Gusher	Starch
Rice Krispies, Kellogg's	Gusher	Starch
shredded wheat, spoonsize	Intermediate	Starch
Shredded Wheat, Post	Gusher	Starch
Smacks, Kellogg's	Intermediate	Starch
Special K, Kellogg's	Trickler	Starch
Team Flakes, Nabisco	Gusher	Starch
Total, General Mills	Gusher	Starch
Weetabix	Gusher	Starch
Breton wheat crackers	Intermediate	Starch
Buckwheat groats, cooked	Trickler	Starch
Bulgur, cooked	Trickler	Starch
Butterbeans (lima), boiled	Trickler	Starch
C		
Cannellini beans, boiled	Trickler	Starch
Cantaloupe, raw	Intermediate	Fruit
Cherries	Trickler	Fruit
Chickpeas		
canned, drained	Trickler	Starch
boiled	Trickler	Starch
Chocolate bar	Trickler	Sugar
Coca-Cola	Intermediate	Sugar
Corn chips	Gusher	Starch
Corn, canned, drained	Intermediate	Starch
Cornmeal, from mix, cooked	Intermediate	Starch
Couscous, cooked	Intermediate	Starch
Crispbread	Gusher	Starch

Food	G.I. Level	Food Category
Croissant, medium	Intermediate	Starch
Custard	Trickler	Starch
D–F		
Dates, dried	Gusher	Fruit
Doughnut with cinnamon and sugar	Gusher	Starch
Fanta	Intermediate	Sugar
Fava beans, frozen, boiled	Gusher	Starch
Flan	Intermediate	Starch
French fries, large	Gusher	Starch
Fructose, pure	Trickler	Sugar
Fruit cocktail, canned in natural juice	Intermediate	Fruit
G		
Gatorade sports drink	Gusher	Sugar
Glucose powder	Gusher	Sugar
Graham crackers	Gusher	Starch
Granola bars, Quaker chewy	Intermediate	Starch
Grapefruit juice, unsweetened	Trickler	Fruit
Grapefruit, raw	Trickler	Fruit
Grapes, green	Trickler	Fruit
Green pea soup, canned, ready to serve	Intermediate	Starch
H–I–J		
Honey	Intermediate	Sugar
Ice cream, 10% fat, vanilla	Intermediate	Dairy, Sugar
Ice milk, vanilla	Trickler	Dairy, Sugar
Jelly beans	Gusher	Sugar
K–L		
Kavli All Natural Whole Grain Crispbread	Gusher	Starch

Food	G.I. Level	Food Category
Kidney beans		
red, boiled	Trickler	Starch
red, canned and drained	Trickler	Starch
Kiwi, medium, raw, peeled	Trickler	Fruit
Kudos Granola Bars (whole-grain)	Intermediate	Starch
Lactose, pure	Trickler	Sugar
Lentil soup, canned	Trickler	Starch
Lentils		
green and brown, boiled	Trickler	Starch
red, boiled	Trickler	Starch
Life Savers, roll candy, peppermint	Gusher	Sugar
Lima beans, baby, frozen	Trickler	Starch
Lychee, canned and drained	Gusher	Fruit
M–N–O		
Macaroni and Cheese Dinner,		
Kraft packaged, cooked	Intermediate	Starch
Maltose (maltodextrin), pure	Gusher	Sugar
Mango	Intermediate	Fruit
Milk		
chocolate flavored, 1%	Trickler	Dairy, Sugar
skim	Trickler	Dairy
whole	Trickler	Dairy
Millet, cooked	Gusher	Starch
Muffins		
apple cinnamon, from mix	Trickler	Starch
apricot and honey, low-fat,		
from mix	Intermediate	Starch
banana, oat, and honey,		
low-fat, from mix	Intermediate	Starch
blueberry	Intermediate	Starch
chocolate butterscotch,		
low-fat, from mix	Trickler	Starch

Food	G.I. Level	Food Category
oat and raisin, low-fat, from mix	Trickler	Starch
oat bran	Intermediate	Starch
Mung beans, boiled	Trickler	Starch
Navy beans, boiled	Trickler	Starch
Nutella (spread)	Trickler	Sugar
Oat bran, raw	Intermediate	Starch
Orange, navel	Trickler	Fruit
P		
Papaya	Intermediate	Fruit
Parsnips, boiled	Gusher	Starch
Pasta		
cappelletti, cooked	Trickler	Starch
fettuccine, cooked	Trickler	Starch
gnocchi, cooked	Intermediate	Starch
linguine, thick, cooked	Trickler	Starch
linguine, thin, cooked	Intermediate	Starch
macaroni, cooked	Trickler	Starch
ravioli, meat-filled, cooked	Trickler	Starch
spaghetti, white, cooked	Trickler	Starch
spaghetti, whole-wheat, cooked	Trickler	Starch
star pastina, cooked	Trickler	Starch
tortellini, cheese, cooked	Trickler	Starch
vermicelli, cooked	Trickler	Starch
Pastry, flaky	Intermediate	Starch
Pea soup, split, with ham	Intermediate	Starch
Peaches		
canned, heavy syrup	Intermediate	Fruit
canned, light syrup	Trickler	Fruit
canned, natural juice	Trickler	Fruit
fresh, 1 medium	Trickler	Fruit

Food	G.I. Level	Food Category
Pears		
canned in pear juice	Trickler	Fruit
fresh	Trickler	Fruit
Peas		
dried, boiled	Trickler	Starch
green, fresh, frozen, boiled	Trickler	Starch
Pineapple, fresh	Intermediate	Fruit
Pinto beans		
canned	Trickler	Starch
soaked, boiled	Trickler	Starch
Pita bread, whole-wheat	Intermediate	Starch
Pizza, cheese and tomato	Intermediate	Starch
Plums	Trickler	Fruit
Popcorn, light, microwave	Intermediate	Starch
Potato chips, plain	Trickler	Starch
Potatoes		
instant mashed, Carnation Foods	Gusher	Starch
new, canned, drained	Intermediate	Starch
new, unpeeled, boiled	Intermediate	Starch
red-skinned, baked in oven (no fat)	Gusher	Starch
red-skinned, mashed	Gusher	Starch
red-skinned, microwaved	Gusher	Starch
red-skinned, peeled, boiled	Gusher	Starch
sweet potato, peeled, boiled	Trickler	Starch
white-skinned, mashed	Intermediate	Starch
white-skinned, peeled, boiled	Intermediate	Starch
white-skinned, with skin, baked in oven (no fat),	Gusher	Starch
white-skinned, with skin, microwaved	Gusher	Starch

Food	G.I. Level	Food Category
Pound cake	Trickler	Starch
Premium saltine crackers	Gusher	Starch
Pretzels	Gusher	Starch
Pudding, cooked	Trickler	Starch
Pumpkin, peeled, boiled, mashed	Gusher	Starch
R		
Raisins	Intermediate	Fruit
Rice bran	Trickler	Starch
Rice cakes, plain	Gusher	Starch
Rice vermicelli, cooked	Intermediate	Starch
Rice		
brown	Intermediate	Starch
basmati, white, boiled	Intermediate	Starch
converted, Uncle Ben's	Trickler	Starch
instant, cooked	Gusher	Starch
long-grain, white	Intermediate	Starch
parboiled	Trickler	Starch
short-grain, white (sticky)	Gusher	Starch
Rutabaga, peeled, boiled	Gusher	Starch
Ryvita tasty dark rye whole-grain		
crisp bread	Intermediate	Starch
S		
Shortbread cookies	Intermediate	Starch
Skittles Original Fruit		
Bite Size Candies	Intermediate	Sugar
Social Tea biscuits, Nabisco	Intermediate	Starch
Soybeans, boiled	Trickler	Starch
Soy milk	Trickler	Dairy
Spirali, durum, cooked	Trickler	Starch
Split pea soup	Intermediate	Starch
Split peas, yellow, boiled	Trickler	Starch
Sponge cake, plain	Trickler	Starch

Food	G.I. Level	Food Category
Stoned wheat thins	Trickler	Starch
Sucrose	Intermediate	Sugar
T–V–W–Y		
Taco shells	Intermediate	Starch
Tomato soup, canned	Trickler	Starch
Twix Chocolate Caramel Cookie	Trickler	Starch
Vanilla wafers	Gusher	Starch
Vitasoy soy milk, creamy original	Trickler	Dairy
Waffles, plain, frozen	Gusher	Starch
Water cracker, Carr's	Gusher	Starch
Watermelon	Gusher	Fruit
Yam, boiled	Trickler	Starch
Yogurt, non-fat		
fruit flavored, artificial sweetener	Trickler	Dairy
fruit flavored, with sugar	Trickler	Dairy
plain, artificial sweetener	Trickler	Dairy

G.I. list reprinted and adapted from *The Glucose Revolution Life Plan,* courtesy of Marlowe & Company.

ACKNOWLEDGMENTS

Hide not your talents, they for use were made.
What's a sun-dial in the shade?
—Benjamin Franklin

- Marie Brown, Laura Garrett, MS, RD, CDE, Barbara Halma, RN, Richard Berkowitz, MD, and Kenneth Lubansky, MD, for generously sharing their thoughts and expertise with me. (J.B.)
- Maria Gill for decades of cooking and sharing recipes with me. (J.B.)
- Lucy and Camille for their unconditional love. (J.B.)
- Ellen Greene for hooking me up with this project.
- Maud, for your thoughtful edits as well as your infinite patience and love. You're my world. (L.R.)
- Matthew Lore, not only for giving us this opportunity, but also for bringing the two of us together.
- The pioneer scientists in Canada and Australia for creating the Glycemic Index, which has helped so many people lead healthier lives. (J.B. and L.R.)

INDEX

ABOUT THE AUTHORS

JOHANNA BURANI, M.S., R.D., C.D.E., is a Registered Dietitian and Certified Diabetes Educator with more than thirteen years' experience in nutritional counseling. The author of several books and professional manuals, including *The Glucose Revolution Life Plan* (with Dr. Jennie Brand-Miller and Kaye Foster-Powell), she specializes in designing individual meal plans based on low-G.I. food choices. She lives in Mendham, New Jersey.

LINDA RAO, M.ED., a freelance writer and editor, has been writing and researching health topics for the past twelve years. Her work has appeared in several national publications, including *Prevention*, *Cooking Light*, and *Health* . She serves as a contributing editor for *Prevention* and lives in Allentown, Pennsylvania.